Clinical Cases in ENT

Clinical Cases in ENT

Geetha Chary MBBS MS DLO
Formerly Professor and Head
Department of ENT
St John's National Academy of Health Sciences
Bengaluru, Karnataka, India

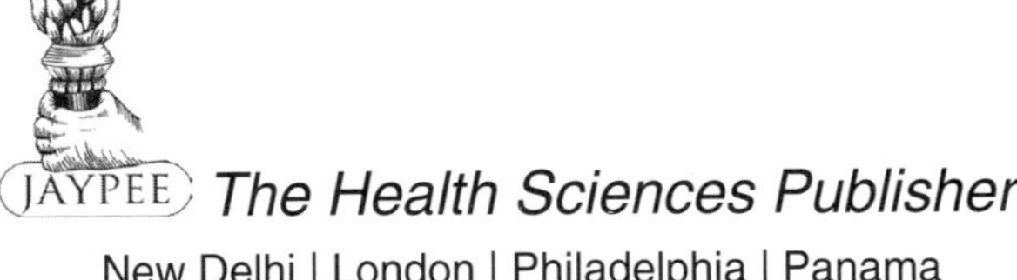

The Health Sciences Publisher
New Delhi | London | Philadelphia | Panama

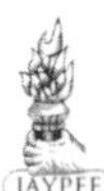

JAYPEE **Jaypee Brothers Medical Publishers (P) Ltd**

Headquarters

Jaypee Brothers Medical Publishers (P) Ltd
4838/24, Ansari Road, Daryaganj
New Delhi 110 002, India
Phone: +91-11-43574357
Fax: +91-11-43574314
Email: jaypee@jaypeebrothers.com

Overseas Offices

J.P. Medical Ltd
83 Victoria Street, London
SW1H 0HW (UK)
Phone: +44 20 3170 8910
Fax: +44 (0)20 3008 6180
Email: info@jpmedpub.com

Jaypee Medical Inc
The Bourse
111 South Independence Mall East
Suite 835, Philadelphia, PA 19106, USA
Phone: +1 267-519-9789
Email: jpmed.us@gmail.com

Jaypee Brothers Medical Publishers (P) Ltd
Bhotahity, Kathmandu, Nepal
Phone: +977-9741283608
Email: kathmandu@jaypeebrothers.com

Jaypee-Highlights Medical Publishers Inc
City of Knowledge, Bld. 237, Clayton
Panama City, Panama
Phone: +1 507-301-0496
Fax: +1 507-301-0499
Email: cservice@jphmedical.com

Jaypee Brothers Medical Publishers (P) Ltd
17/1-B Babar Road, Block-B, Shaymali
Mohammadpur, Dhaka-1207
Bangladesh
Mobile: +08801912003485
Email: jaypeedhaka@gmail.com

Website: www.jaypeebrothers.com
Website: www.jaypeedigital.com

Inquiries for bulk sales may be solicited at: jaypee@jaypeebrothers.com

Clinical Cases in ENT

First Edition: **2015**

ISBN: 978-93-5152-726-8

Printed at Rajkamal Electric Press, Plot No. 2, Phase-IV, Kundli, Haryana.

PREFACE

This book has been written to give the postgraduate (PG) students a comprehensive idea of what to look for in patients who routinely visit the hospital.

There is an emphasis on history-taking, because good history accomplishes more than half the job. Routine clinical examination done in a systematic manner reveals a lot of information. There are instances when a thyroid swelling, for example, is seen from a distance and sent for fine needle aspiration cytology (FNAC)/thyroid function test. Arriving at a clinical diagnosis before investigating is invaluable. To this end, clinical examination has been described in some detail.

This book could be a ready reckoner prior to the PG clinical examination as it deals with cases usually given in such examinations.

I am sure, general practitioners and ENT consultants will find this book useful in their routine clinical work.

All the material in this book is what I have gained from my teachers and the textbooks. I would like to acknowledge all my teachers. Postgraduate students and their weekly case presentations have contributed in a big way to this book.

My thanks to all my colleagues in ENT, for sharing their clinical experiences and the dilemmas faced when treating patients.

Last but not least, I would like to thank my family, for their constant support in my life.

Geetha Chary

CONTENTS

Chapter 1:	**Chronic Otitis Media**	**1**
Chapter 2:	**Chronic Otitis Media with Cholesteatoma**	**20**
Chapter 3:	**Facial Nerve Palsy**	**27**
Chapter 4:	**Vertigo**	**34**
Chapter 5:	**Hard of Hearing**	**41**
Chapter 6:	**Deviated Nasal Septum**	**49**
Chapter 7:	**Sinonasal Polyps**	**57**
Chapter 8:	**Inverted Papilloma**	**66**
Chapter 9:	**Sinonasal Malignancy**	**71**
Chapter 10:	**Nasopharyngeal Angiofibroma**	**80**
Chapter 11:	**Nasopharyngeal Carcinoma**	**85**
Chapter 12:	**Oral Cavity**	**94**
Chapter 13:	**Oropharyngeal Mass**	**105**
Chapter 14:	**Vocal Nodules**	**116**
Chapter 15:	**Left Vocal Cord Paralysis**	**125**
Chapter 16:	**Supraglottic Carcinoma**	**130**
Chapter 17:	**Glottic Cancer**	**139**
Chapter 18:	**Laryngopharyngeal Carcinoma**	**148**
Chapter 19:	**Thyroid Neoplasm**	**157**
Chapter 20:	**Goiter**	**172**
Chapter 21:	**Thyroglossal Cyst**	**178**
Chapter 22:	**Parotid Swelling**	**180**
Chapter 23:	**Submandibular Gland Swelling**	**189**
Chapter 24:	**Cervical Lymphadenopathy with Unknown Primary**	**195**
Index		*205*

Chapter 1

Chronic Otitis Media

A 23-year-old girl presents with history of ear discharge both ears since childhood. History of pain in the right ear since 1 week.

HISTORY OF PRESENT ILLNESS

Pain in the right ear started one week ago. It was very severe and she went to a family physician who prescribed tablets and ear drops. She was advised by the doctor to see an ENT specialist for her discharge.

- *Otalgia is a symptom of external auditory canal disease:*

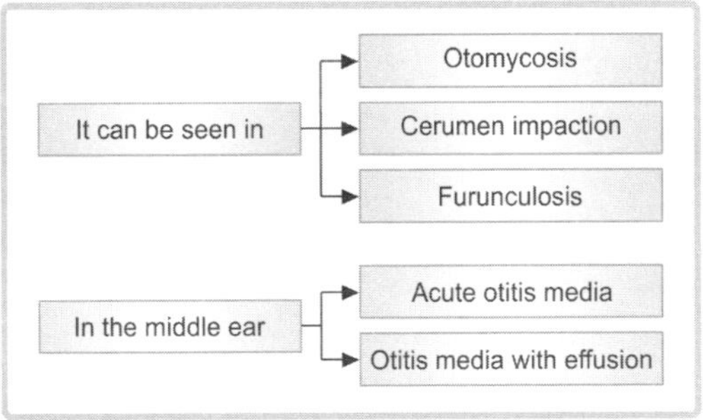

  - *In chronic otitis media, pain is associated with external canal infection or complications*
  - *Referred pain in the ear is usually due to pathology in the aerodigestive tract*
  - *Pain can also be due to temperomandibular joint disease*
  - The discharge in both the ears is profuse, mucoid and intermittent. It is not foul smelling or blood stained. Discharge increases when she has nasal block/nasal discharge/throat pain/or when water enters the ear.
- *Ear discharge can be watery as in CSF otorrhea.*
  - *Discharge is scanty if external canal is infected or in infections of areas of the middle ear cleft which are not lined by respiratory type of epithelium*
  - *If ear discharge is profuse, the epithelium involved is pseudostratified ciliated columnar epithelium which has mucous producing glands and goblet cells*

- *Foul smelling discharge is seen in anaerobic infections*
- *Blood stained discharge is seen in patients with granulation tissue formation. Granulation tissue occurs due to osteitis.*

She says her mother told her that as a child of 1½ years she had severe ear pain once and it was followed by ear discharge which relieved the pain. Since then the ear has been discharging on and off. She used ear drops and of late the discharge has reduced in amount and frequency. She has no history of hard of hearing.

- Hard of hearing
  - Patient has no hard of hearing.
  - *If patient has hearing loss it can be:*

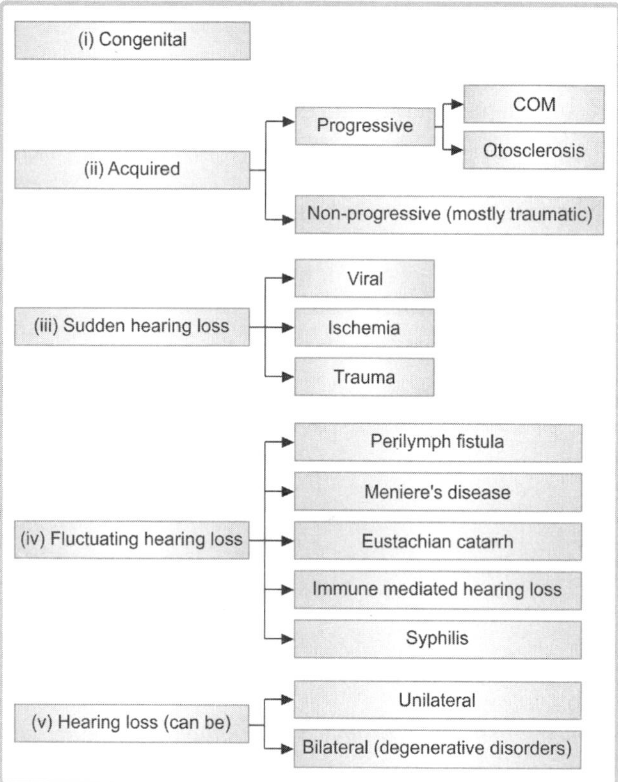

- *So, the questions to be asked are:*
  1. Is it congenital or acquired?
  2. Is it progressive?
  3. Has there been trauma (physical and noise)?
  4. Was there fever?
  5. Is there an intake of drugs (some medication can cause deafness)?
  6. Is the hearing loss fluctuating?

7. It is unilateral or bilateral?
8. Are there any other associated ear symptoms?
9. Is there family history of deafness (otosclerosis)?
10. What is the patient's occupation?

Hearing loss in children can be due to prenatal, postnatal, or perinatal causes. Look for syndromic association.

Commonest genetic mutation is connexin 26 (nonsyndromic).

- Vertigo
  - Patient has no history of vertigo.
  - *If patient has history of vertigo, the questions to be asked are:*

1. *How long does it last?*
   Less than a minute (benign positional vertigo)
   A few minutes (migrainous vertigo)
   A few hours (Meniere's disease)
   A few days (vestibular neuronitis)
2. *Do you feel you are rotating or is the room rotating?*
   In true vertigo the room and its objects rotate.
   (Vertigo is a false sense of orientation of oneself to one's surroundings)
3. *Is it associated with deafness?*

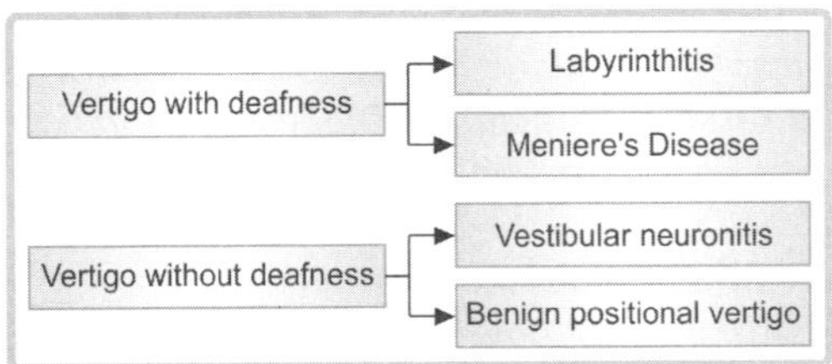

4. *Is it associated with ear discharge?*
   If it is associated with ear discharge, it may be labyrinthitis/fistula in the lateral semicircular canal.
   Is it episodic?
   Meniere's disease
6. *Is it brought on by alteration in head or body position?*
   Benign positional vertigo
   Orthostatic vertigo
7. *Is there history of migraine?*
8. *Is there syncope?*
   Peripheral vertigo is not associated with syncope.
9. *Has it lasted for more than 6 weeks?*
   After 3 weeks of vertigo of peripheral origin compensation occurs.
10. *Are you on any long-term drugs?*
    Anti-hypertensive and anti-depressants can cause a sense of unsteadiness.

- Tinnitus

Do you have tinnitus?

No.

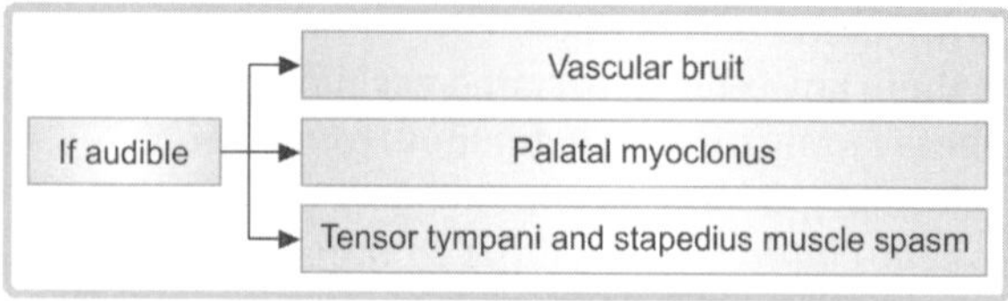

Non audible tinnitus is mostly seen in sensorineural loss.
No history of loss of consciousness, headache, fever, or irritability.
(This occurs due to intracranial complications)
History of nasal obstruction right side present all the time.
No history of nasal discharge/sneezing/anosmia/epistaxis.
Patient has no history of previous surgical treatment and has undergone medical treatment for ear discharge.
No previous history of investigations such as imaging/PTA. etc.
No history of allergy to medication.

PAST HISTORY

No past history of diabetes, renal disease, thyroid disease, or tuberculosis.

Ear problems in diabetes: Furunculosis, otomycosis, malignant otitis externa, multiple cranial nerve palsies due to diabetic neuropathy usually III cranial nerve, but VII and VIII can be involved. Diabetes does not cause sensorineural loss per se but is involved in some syndromes where diabetes occurs with hearing loss.

Renal system can be involved along with auditory system in hereditary syndromes such as Alports and some drugs cause nephrotoxicity and ototoxicity.

Thyroid disease: Goiters can be associated with sensorineural loss (Pendreds syndrome).

Tuberculosis can cause otitis media.

Socioeconomic status/number of siblings has an impact on ear disease in children as upper respiratory tract infection can cause otitis media with effusion/acute otitis media (OME/AOM).

From the history it appears to be chronic otitis media of the mucosal type because of profuse and intermittent discharge which is not foul smelling or blood stained with no complications.

How did it start?

There is a history of AOM in childhood.

What is the pain due to?

Pain may be due to otitis externa.

Why is there no hearing loss?

The hearing loss may not be perceived as a disability by the patient.

General Examination

- Patient is conscious, well-oriented to time, place and person
- Moderately built and nourished
- No pallor, icterus, cyanosis, clubbing, generalized lymphadenopathy or pedal edema
- Pulse 72/minute, BP 120/80
- Respiratory rate 18 per minute
- CVS: NAD (no abnormality detected)
- RS: NAD
- Abdomen: NAD
- CNS and cranial nerves: normal except VIII.

Fever

- *Brain abscess; low grade fever in stage one (encephalitis)*
- *Lateral sinus thrombosis: Picket fence fever/but when modified due to antibiotics it can be high grade fever which does not reach the base line*
- *Meningitis: High grade fever.*

Pulse

- *Brain abscess: slow pulse in the late stages*
- *Meningitis (proportionate to fever)*
- *Lateral sinus thrombosis (proportionate to fever).*

ENT EXAMINATION

Right ear: Pinna is normal.

Look for cellulitis, erythema, dermatitis, neoplasm, and deformities.

Pinna can be pushed forward due to furunculosis.

Pinna is yellow elastic cartilage and has helix, anti helix, tragus, well of ear. Lobule has no cartilage. Pinna does not ossify because yellow elastic cartilage does not ossify.

Pulling the pinna backwards or pressure once tragus causes pain in furunculosis.

Pressure over the tragus can cause Tullio phenomenon (vertigo). This is seen is superior semicircular canal dehiscence.

Preauricular region-normal.

Look for scar's, sinus, lymph node and skin tags.

Postauricular region-normal.

Scar in the postaural region can be postoperative. Swelling may be due to mastoid abscess/furunculosis. Postauricular groove is preserved in mastoid abscess where as in furunculosis it is obliterated. This is because pus is below the periosteum in mastoiditis.

Well of the ear is normal.

Vesicles are seen in the well of the ear in herpes zoster oticus.

External auditory canal: There are whitish debris on the floor. No other abnormality seen. No pus seen.

Whitish debris are seen in candidiasis, they appear like wet blotting paper.

Whitish debris with black spots indicates aspergillus niger, this looks like wet newspaper.

Dark brown material in the external canal is usually wax.

Wax is colorless when secreted and is a combination of secretions of sweat and sebaceous glands and it becomes brown due to oxidation.

Desquamated epithelium and debris may also be seen in the external canal.

Length of external canal is 2.5 cm (tympanic membrane is situated beyond this). It is not straight and pinna has to be pulled upwards and backwards to visualize tympanic membrane.

Fissures of Santorini in the cartilaginous part of the external canal allow pus to reach parotid space and vice versa.

External canal can show:

- *Stenosis*
  - *Traumatic*
  - *Congenital*
- *Cellulitis*
- *Furunculosis*
- *Cysts*
- *Edema*
- *Dermatitis*
- *Exposed bone (external auditory canal cholesteatoma)*
- *Widening (keratosis obturans)*
- *Granulations at the junction of cartilaginous and bony canal (skull base osteomyelitis) Granulations are also seen in COM*
- *Sagging of posterior meatal wall is seen in coalescent mastoiditis.*
- *Aural polyp*
  - *COM*
  - *Glomus jugulare*
  - *Schwannomas.*

Is the polyp arising from the external canal or middle ear?

In external canal polyp probe cannot be passed all around.

- *In canal wall down mastoidectomy cavity can be seen, look for—*
  - *Recurrent cholesteatoma*
  - *Size of meatoplasty*
  - *Probable surgical problems such as high facial ridge, granulations, fungus and wax in the cavity.*
- Examination of tympanic membrane:
  - Color: normal
  - *Normal color is gray and translucent*
  - *Normal structures seen are handle of malleus, cone of light in the antero-inferior quadrant, posterior and anterior malleolar folds, shadow*

of long process of incus, lateral process of malleus, pars tensa and pars flaccida.

Abnormalities

Perforation can be in the pars tensa/pars flaccida/posterior margin. A central perforation is a perforation of the pars tensa with a rim of drum all around. This can be large, small or pinhole size. It can involve all quadrants of the pars tensa (anterior, inferior and posterior). It can be subtotal.

Edges of the perforation can be hyperemic or pale.

Why do perforations occur in the posterior margin?

- Perforations occur in the posterior margin because there is a lease of vessels to the posterior margin and so inflammatory processes are accentuated and result in a perforation here
- Thinned out area of the drum due to healed drum (dimeric membrane)
- Tympanic membrane may be retracted
- Pars tensa retraction (Sade's):
  - Grade I slight retraction of tympanic membrane (retraction)
  - Grade II Tympanic membrane touching incus or stapes (severe retraction)
  - Grade III Tympanic membrane touches promontory (atelectasis)
  - Grade IV Tympanic membrane adherent to promontory (adhesive otitis). Of these Grade I–III are reversible, but Grade IV is not reversible.

What are the signs of retraction?

- Loss or distortion of cone of light
- Prominent or fore shortening of handle of malleus
- Prominent anterior and posterior malleolar folds
- Long process of incus seen through the drum/draping of tympanic membrane on the long process of incus or incudo stapedial joint.

What are the grades of pars flaccida retraction (Tos's)?

- Stage I pars flaccida is dimpled and more retracted than normal but is not adherent to malleus
- Stage II retraction is adherent to neck of malleus but retraction pocket is well seen.
- Stage III retraction is out of view and partial erosion of scutum
- Stage IV definite erosion of outer attic wall and retraction pocket out of view
- Stage III and IV are somewhat similar.

Tympanosclerotic patches may be seen on the tympanic membrane. Grommet insertion causes a typical crescent shaped tympanosclerotic patch.

What are the structures seen through a perforation?

- Mucosa over promontory
- Eustachian tube orifice
- Incudostapedial joint
- Parts of hypotympanum
- Attic.

Mobility of tympanic membrane can be tested by pneumatic otoscopy.

What are the uses of pneumatic otoscopy?

- Mobility of drum
- Middle ear fluid (when pressure is increased serous fluid sticks to the drum)
- To distinguish between tympanosclerosis of tympanic membrane from middle ear tympanosclerosis
- Retraction pockets
- Atelectatic process
- Fistula test
- Can also be used to push ear drops into middle ear
- Provides magnification of 1.5 diopters.

What is the differential diagnosis for a vascular mass seen behind tympanic membrane?

- Dehiscent jugular bulb
- Aberrant internal carotid artery
- Glomus jugular
- Middle ear tumors
- Aneurysm.

What is the differential diagnosis for a white mass seen behind tympanic membrane?

- Purulent debris
- Cholesteatoma
- Tympano sclerosis
- Middle ear avascular mass
- Fused ossicular chain.

In this patient

Right ear: central perforation in the pars tensa involving inferior and anterior quadrants. Rest of pars tensa normal.

- No cholesteatoma flakes seen.
- No granulation tissue seen.
- Middle ear mucosa appears normal.
- Handle of malleus seen through the perforation.
- Tympanic membrane is mobile.

Left ear: pinna, pre and postauricular regions are normal. External auditory canal no pus or debris seen.

A central perforation involving anterior and inferior quadrant seen, smaller in size when compared to right ear. Middle ear mucosa is normal, handle of malleus seen, no other middle ear structures seen.

No mastoid tenderness:

Mastoid tenderness is elicited over bony areas around antrum. 3-point tenderness refers to placing a finger in the well of the ear, one in the post auricular region over Mac Ewan's triangle and a third on the mastoid tip. Mastoid tenderness is seen in acute coalescent mastoiditis.

Describe tuning fork test:

Rinnes test—differentiate between normal, conductive and sensorineural loss. Usually done using 256, 512, 1024; even though 512 is used more frequently, 256 has greater sensitivity and specificity.

Tuning fork is struck on the elbow, if struck on a harder surface it produces overtones. A struck tuning fork has 70 dB intensity.

Threshold comparison test—hold an activated tuning fork in front of the external canal and when patient stops place it over the mastoid.

Relative loudness test—alternate the activated tuning fork between external canal and mastoid and ask patient to say which is louder. This is more sensitive.

In normal ears air conduction is better than bone conduction.

Sensorineural loss—air conduction is better than bone but it is reduced.

Conductive hearing loss—bone conduction is better than air conduction called negative Rinne.

False negative Rinne—if for example the patient has sensorineural loss in the right ear, when the tuning fork is held in front of the right ear he cannot hear but he perceives sound when fork is placed over mastoid. This is because when fork is placed on the mastoid sound travels to the opposite ear through the skull bones. So it appears as if bone conduction is better than air but it is really not so.

Weber's test—is not so sensitive or specific. It gives result only if one already knows which is the better and worse ear by other tests.

Activated tuning fork is placed over forehead, nasion or central incisors and patient is asked to say which side he hears.

Normal—heard equally in both ears

Conductive loss lateralized to worse ear.

Sensorineural loss lateralized to better ear.

Absolute bone conduction—An activated tuning fork is placed on the mastoid process of the patient while the external canal is closed with tragus. When he stops hearing it is transferred to the mastoid process of the examiner whose external canal is closed with tragus. If examiner hears after patient stops hearing than patients ABC is reduced indicating senosorineural hearing loss. This assumes that the examiner has normal hearing.

In the absence of audiometry, how can the degree of conductive hearing loss be assessed?

By doing the Rinne's test with all three tuning forks.

If Rinne is negative for 256, but positive for 512;, then A-B gap is 20 to 30 dB.

If Rinne is negative for 256 and 512, but positive for 1024; then A-B gap is 30 to 40 dB.

If Rinne is negative for all three tuning forks; then A-B gap is 45 to 60 dB.

Which is the more sensitive test, Weber or Rinne?

In conductive loss Weber is lateralized if loss is 5-8 dB and Rinne is negative if hearing loss is 15-20 dB.

This patient has:

	Right	*Left*
Rinne	Negative	Negative
Weber	Lateralized to right	
ABC	Not reduced	Not reduced

She has bilateral conductive loss and the right ear is worse.

Tests for vestibular function:-

- Fistula test negative
- Describe Fistula test.

Fistula test: can be done using Siegle's pneumatic speculum or by alternating pressure in the external canal by pressing and releasing the tragus repeatedly.

Patient may experience vertigo and nystagmus may be seen and this is a positive fistula sign.

Positive fistula test:

- Lateral semicircular canal fistula
- Oval or round window fistula
- Perilymph fistula/post stapedectomy
- Labyrinthitis.

  If fistula test is negative but fistula is present (false negative fistula sign)
  Seen in dead labyrinth/or if fistula is covered with cholesteatoma matrix
  If fistula test is positive but there is no fistula (false positive fistula sign) (Hennebert's sign)
  Meniere's disease (saccule is distended and is in contact with oval window)

Syphilis: Here also there is endolymphatic hydrops.

In fistula sign compression nystagmus occurs to diseased side, slow component to opposite side. Whereas in reverse fistula sign slow component is towards diseased side. This reverse fistula sign is seen in hyper mobile stapes.

- Look for spontaneous nystagmus. Patient has no spontaneous nystagmus. Describe spontaneous nystagmus. This occurs due to imbalance between inputs from both labyrinths. It is usually seen in unilateral lesions and in acute vestibular failure. If nystagmus is seen only when one eye is closed it is usually congenital and abnormally present OKN in such cases can be ignored.

- If nystagmus is present on tragal pressure or valsalva it is usually due to superior semicircular canal dehiscence
- Vestibular nystagmus is usually horizontal has a slow and fast component and is named after the fast component. It has a latent period and is fatigable, for example: if right vestibule is hypoactive then brain receives information from left and not right. It imagines head is turned to right. The correcting component moves eyes to left and this is the fast component
- Vestibular nystagmus disappears on visual fixation. Three grades are:
    1. Grade I when patient looks towards fast component
    2. Grade II when patient looks straight
    3. Grade III when patient looks towards slow component.

Alexander's law: A second or third-degree nystagmus will enhance on looking towards fast component.

In later stages (after acute phase of vestibular failure is over) only gaze induced nystagmus can be elicited.

- Gaze evoked induced nystagmus: Patient has no gaze induced nystagmus
  Describe gaze induced nystagmus:
    - If spontaneous nystagmus is absent look for gaze induced nystagmus. This is present after the acute phase of vestibular failure is over.
    - Move the finger in front of the patient towards the right and left slowly. Nystagmus may be induced with a slow and fast component.
    - This gaze evoked nystagmus must be differentiated from gaze paretic nystagmus due to central lesion. In a right-sided central lesion (cerebellum and brain stem involvement) when patient looks to the extreme right (eccentric position) the gaze cannot be held and eye slowly drifts to the centre and a saccade is needed to refix eye eccentrically. Here nystagmus (fast component) is towards lesion side unlike gaze induced nystagmus where nystagmus is towards opposite side.
    - If there is a VIII N tumor involving peripheral vestibular system and brain stem both gaze evoked and gaze paretic nystagmus will be present known as Brun's nystagmus.
- Head thrust test: No saccades seen
  Describe head thrust test:
    - Place patients head slightly over midline (say to the right) and rotate head rapidly either by examiner or patient himself and nystagmus is looked for. When testing left labyrinth turn head briskly to the opposite side. Patients eyes should be fixed on an object. If vestibule is functioning, eye will remain fixed on the object. In acute unilateral vestibular failure eye will not remain fixed and there will be saccades to fix it back.
    - A right head turn in a person with acute right vestibular failure will result in catch up saccades to the left.

- Normally no saccades are seen. In unilateral acute dysfunction there are saccades with component towards uninvolved side. In chronic lesion the test is inconclusive.
- This test differentiates between acute vestibular failure and central causes in the emergency room.

- Examination of cranial nerves normal
- Cerebellar function tests normal
  - Cerebellar function tests such as finger nose test, flipping palm on base of hand alternatively (dysdiadochokinesia)
  - *Heel to toe test:* There is incoordination in cerebellar lesions. In vestibular failure, patient falls towards involved side.
- Romberg's test normal
  Describe Romberg's test: Romberg's test examines vestibulo spinal tract. Patient stands erect with feet together both with eyes open and closed. He falls to the side of uncompensated involved labyrinth. This can also be done with patient's arms folded over chest which is a sharpened Romberg's test and is more sensitive.
- Untenberger's test normal
  Describe Untenberger's test: In Untenberger's test patient marches in a place with eyes closed and arms outstretched and clasped together anteriorly. Body rotation of more than 30° or backward and forward displacement of 1 meter is abnormal. Having patient step on 6" foam eliminates proprioception. (Fukuda stepping test is similar).
- Positional test normal.

Dix-hallpike Maneuver : No nystagmus seen

Describe Dix-hallpike maneuver: Patient sits on a couch and his head is turned 45° to the right and then patient is made supine with head hanging. This makes the movement in the plane of right posterior semicircular canal. Keep patient in this position for a few seconds as there is a long latency. Next bring back patient to sitting position, turn head to left at 45° and make the patient supine. This maneuver results in a positional nystagmus. If done on left side the upper pole of left eye beats towards left shoulder. This is followed by an upbeating nystagmus which is also seen synchronous with tortional nystagmus. Patient also experiences intense vertigo and may try to sit up. Patient otherwise has normal vestibular function.

In patients with cervical spondylitis the same test can be done without hanging the head off the couch. (Bojrate-Calvert maneuver).

Fundoscopy normal.

Fundoscopy is done to rule out raised intracranial tension.

Auscultate neck for bruit (Carotid bifurcation).

Examination of nose and PNS: No abnormality seen except deviated septum to the right.

Diagnosis: Chronic oti tis media both ears. Inactive mucosal disease with bilateral conductive loss worse on the right side with no complications.

What are the types of mucosal chronic otitis media?

- Healed mucosal disease; end result is a dimeric membrane or tympanosclerotic patch
- Inactive disease, where a dry central perforation is present
- Active mucosal disease where
  - Perforation
  - Pus
  - Parts of ossicular chain seen eroded
  - Polyp
  - Granulation tissue.

Can you classify safe and unsafe ear depending on site of perforation?

Site of perforation does not make ear safe or unsafe. It is true that an attic or posterior marginal perforation is more prone to have cholesteatoma and hence complications. Even granulation tissue can cause intracranial complications irrespective of whether cholesteatoma is present or not. Both cholesteatoma and granulation tissue cause bony erosion.

How will you investigate this patient?

- Examination under the microscope:
  - Look for size, shape and position of perforation
  - Look at the margin of the perforation to see where the squamous epithelium meets the mucosal layer
  - Look for the color of middle ear mucosa (pale, edematous, red)
  - Look for granulations, polyps
  - Parts of ossicular chain may be seen such as handle of malleus , incudostapedial joint
  - Look for dimeric drum, tympanoscerotic patches.
- Culture and sensitivity if discharge is present.
  In this patient, there is no discharge.

Most common organism—pseudomonas aeroginose. It penetrates host system by producing proteases, lipases which initiate local immunological system and allow colonization. It forms a biofilm.

Other organisms are *Staphylococcus aureus,* diptheroids, streptococci, gram-negative bacilli such as *Proteus mirabalis,* anaerobes and fungi are also present. Bacteroides and fusiform bacterium can also be seen.

Synergy between anaerobes and aerobes increases incidence and such mixed infections are seen in intracranial complications.

How do you take an ear swab for culture and sensitivity?

To avoid contamination from external auditory canal organisms an insulin or tuberculin syringe is used to collect material from the middle ear without touching walls of external canal.

What are biofilms?

Biofilms refer to a matrix of polysaccharides formed by colonies of bacteria. This matrix protects the bacteria and helps it to survive. The polysaccharides coat the surface of a colony of the bacteria. The biofilm prevents destruction of organism by antibiotics and immune system. When swabs are taken for culture and sensitivity it is negative as bacteria are sequestered on the surface of lining mucosa.

The bacteria secretes exo and endotoxin which initiates an inflammatory process. Of all factors TNF α and IL-1b are responsible for mastoid and middle ear infections. Both are secreted by macrophages. Inflammatory mediators thicken mucosa by causing mucosal layer differentiation into goblet cells and ciliated cells.

Are organisms responsible for persistent COM?

Elimination of an aerobes does not heal COM. So there is a primary inflammatory process where bacteria are secondary invaders.

- Pure tone audiometry

  It gives a qualitative and quantitative assessment of hearing loss.

What does air bone gap depend on?

- Size of perforation, large perforation opens round window to atmosphere
- Erosion of ossicular chain
- Significant granulations around ossicular chain.

What is masking?

If air conduction loss is asymmetrical in two ears by 40 dB then when the worse ear is tested by air conduction vibratory noise is carried to contralateral cochlea through the skull. So, bone conduction should be masked. Masking noise is presented to determine first audible level and then raised by 5 dB.

How is pure tone audiometry (PTA) done?

Sound is increased from inaudible to audible in 5 dB sounds. As soon as he hears it is decreased by 10 dB and again increased by 5 dB onwards. Three correct responses to 3–5 ascending stimuli series is taken as the threshold for that frequency. First 1000 Hz is tested, then higher frequency followed by the lowest. Frequencies tested are 250, 500, 1,000, 2,000 and 4,000.

Alternatively ascend and then descend at same 5 dB. The average of 3 lowest audible ascent and 3 lowest audible descent is the threshold.

What is audiometric zero?

Audiometric zero or 0 dB hearing loss is the average intensity level at which threshold is measured in normal hearing individuals.

What is speech audiometry?

Speech audiometry starts at 20-30 dB above pure tone audiometry (PTA) at 500, 1000, 2000 Hz. Then it is reduced by 5 dB levels, 10 test items are presented. At least 50% should be correct. Then it is tested by 10 items at 5 dB lower level. Speech reception threshold is calculated from the data 50% of words heard at the lowest level and highest level that yielded less than 50% correct response.

Maximum speech reception score: Phonetically balanced words at 20-25 dB above speech recognition threshold (SRT) are presented and then increased by 5 dB till 100% of speech is heard. If on reaching high level there is a decrease in the score it is due to roll over effect. Then bring it down to lower level.

PTA = SRT normal/conductive hearing loss
PTA > SRT retrocochlear deafness
PTA < SRT malingerer

In retrocochlear deafness, speech discrimination is lost disproportionate to hearing loss.

What is a decibel?

- Auditory system operates over a wide range of stimulus intensities
- So, a lograthamic scale is used to measure it
- Decibel is the ratio of the amplitude of measured sound to a reference sound
- In audiology, sound is measured as sound pressure levels (SPL)
- The reference sound has a SPL of 0.0002 dynes/cm^2 which corresponds to the threshold of hearing in normal subjects at 1000 Hz
- Decibel is 1/10th of a bell
- The SPL range can be 0.0002 dynes/cm^2 at normal thresholds to 200 dynes/cm^2 which can cause pain. If a sound has an SPL of 1000, i.e. 10^3 times the reference sound, then it is expressed as 20 x 3 = 60 dB; because the formula used to calculate is:
  20 log (SPL of S_1/SPL of S_2) where S_2 is the reference sound and S_1 is the sound being measured.

X-ray both mastoids: Schullers view where X-ray beam is projected 30º cepalocaudal is better than Laws view which is 15º cepalocaudal, as it prevents super imposition of both mastoids.

Both mastoids taken for the following reasons:

- Types of mastoid
  - Cellular
  - Sclerotic
  - Diploeic.

  80% of human beings are born with cellular mastoids.

  Cells of the mastoid are antrum (largest cell and most likely to be present). Periantral cells, facial nerve cells, cells along dura, sinus plate, tip cells, petrous cells, zygomatic cells.
  - Low lying dura
  - Forward placed sinus

- Cavity in the mastoid may be due to
  - Cholesteatoma
  - Large antrum
  - Large cell
  - Operated cavity
  - Eosinoptial granuloma
  - Tumors
  - Tuberculosis.

  Cholesteatoma cavity has a rim of sclerotic bone around it unlike operated cavity.

CT scan—1.5 mm cuts in axial and coronal planes.

When will you do a CT scan?

- When otomicroscopy does not give conclusive results
- When symptoms persist in an otherwise normal tympanic membrane
- When congenital cholesteatoma is suspected
- Revision surgery
- When complications intracranial or intratemporal are present
  It is 83% false positive for fistula
- When operating on the only hearing ear
  Cholesteatoma is seen as a soft tissue density
- MRI .

In MRI, cholesteatoma is seen as low intensity on T_1 and high on T_2 weighted images; but it cannot be differentiated from other inflammatory conditions.

What causes COM and its persistence?

- Biofilms
- Acute otitis media
- Eustachian tube dysfunction
- Permanent perforation
- Tympanostomy tubes
- Low socioeconomic status (day care, prematurity, lack of breast feeding are predisposing factors for acute otitis media)
- Entry of water into ear
- Mastoid infection.

How will you treat this patient?

As it is inactive COM both ears the peforation can be grafted with temporalis fascia.

Why is temporalis fascia used and are there other materials that can be used?

Temporalis fascia is available at the site of operation and it has the same BMR as the tympanic membrane. Other materials such as tragal perichondrium can also be used.

What is myringoplasty?

Repair of the drum is known as myringoplasty. It can be done using overlay or underlay technique through a postaural incision, the skin of external auditory canal is elevated till it reaches the annulus which is also elevated. Prior to grafting, the rim of drum should be freshened because squamous epithelial has grown inwards to fuse with the mucosal lining and hence healing has not occurred. All squamous epithelium along handle of malleus should be removed and the graft placed beneath annulus and handle of malleus. In case of a large perforation the graft can be tucked anteriorly below annulus and anterior canal skin. This is the underlay technique. Overlay technique involves placing the graft over the drum through a transcanal approach.

What are the factors affecting graft uptake?

- Size of perforation (in smaller perforation, take is better)
- Expertise of surgeon
- Improvement in hearing is 8 dB
- Preoperative antibiotics does not make a difference
- Takes up even if ear is wet.

How do you know you are competent to do a myringoplasty?

At least 56% of your cases should have graft uptake.

What happens to the graft following myringoplasty?

The graft becomes the middle layer of the drum and squamous epithelium grows over it laterally and mucosa covers it medially.

Which ear will you operate on?

The ear with worse hearing loss or the one with larger perforation if hearing loss is same on both sides.

If everything is equal (size of perforation/hearing loss) the ear which the patient prefers should be operated on.

What are the complications of myringoplasty?

- Non uptake of graft
- Graft lateralization (graft should be in contact with rim)
- Graft medialization (injury to medial wall of middle ear causing adhesion)
- Reperforation of graft
- Residual perforation
- Transient facial palsy due to local anesthesia may be because of dehiscent facial canal
- Graft uptake is better in older children than younger children
- Anterior blunting when the angulation between the canal wall and drum is lost

- Epithelial pearl formation (all squamous epithelium such as epithelium on the edge of perforation,on the handle of malleus, and medial surface of the drum has to be removed from the middle ear before grafting).

If ear is discharging, what will be your treatment?

- Patient can be told to keep ear dry by using a cotton wick soaked in vaseline during bathing
- Antibiotic ear drops such as ciprofloxacin or oflaxacin can be used
- Systemic antibiotics do not hasten the process of infection control
- Antiseptic ear drops are as effective as antibiotic ear drops
- Upper respiratory tract infection can be controlled medically/surgically
- If ear is still discharging a canal wall up mastoid exploration can be done.

What are the indications for canal wall up mastoidectomy (cortical mastoidectomy)?

(This is also called simple mastoidectomy/Schwartz's mastoidectomy).

- COM mucosal type not healed by medical treatment
- COM of squamosal type when it can be combined with posterior tympanotomy and atticotomy
- It is sometimes done in otitis media with effusion along with myringotomy and grommet insertion
- In acute coalescent mastoiditis/masked mastoiditis
- As an approach to facial nerve decompression
- As an approach to endolymphatic sac
- As an approach to cochleostomy during cochlear implant
- As an approach to the labyrinth, internal acoustic meatus and skull base.

Describe cortical mastoidectomy

The mastoid is opened through a postaural incision made 1 cm from the post aural groove. The bone over the Mac Evan's triangle is drilled because the mastoid antrum lies 1.5 cm deep to the triangle. The triangle is formed by the supramastoid crest, posterior meatal wall and a tangential line connecting the two. The Mac Evan's triangle can also be identified by the cribriform nature of its bone and by a spicule of bone anteriorly called spine of Henle. Once antrum is reached all air cells are exenterated and saucerization of mastoid is done. The bony landmarks to indication complete saucerization are superiorly tegmen plate is seen and posteriorly sigmoid sinus plate and inferiorly digastric ridge is visible.

Complications

- Facial nerve paralysis due to
  - Local anesthetic agents (transient)
  - Heat of drill
  - Dehiscent facial canal driving a spicule of bone on to facial nerve
- Bleeding over sigmoid sinus can be controlled with bipolar cautery

- Injury to dura
- Subluxation of incus
- Traumatic high tone loss (is seen particularly in children).

Following cortical mastoidectomy, myringoplasty can be done. If there is ossicular discontinuity/ossiculoplasty.

What is Korner's septum?

It is an embryological remnant of bony plate between petrous and squamous bone which can cause difficulty in approaching antrum through a postaural approach. It separates superficial squamous cells from deeper petrosal cells. Mastoid antrum entry is possible only after removal of the septum as antrum is deep to it.

Chapter 2

Chronic Otitis Media with Cholesteatoma

A 45-year-old man who is a teacher by occupation presents in the outpatient with blood stained ear discharge right ear—1 weeks duration.

HISTORY OF PRESENT ILLNESS

Patient noticed that the right ear discharge which he has been having since one year has become blood stained over the past week. The discharge in the right ear has been small in quantity, foul smelling. He has been undergoing treatment for the same with tablets and ear drops from a family physician. The discharge has never been blood stained before and this made him seek a specialist opinion. The discharge has no relation to upper respiratory tract infection and is continuous.

He is hard of hearing since 6 months and this has been progressive. He is finding it difficult to place which child is speaking to him in class.
(Binaural hearing is essential for localization of sound)
(All of history of for deafness as in chapter 1)
No history of vertigo
No history of tinnitus
No history of otalgia

Ask all other history as in chapter 1.
No other positive history.

Not a smoker or alcoholic:
(smoking and passive smoking can cause ciliary dysfunction and result in otitis media with effusion especially in young children with parents who smoke).

From the history it appears to be chronic otitis media of the squamosal type in the right ear with hearing impairment and no other complications.
General examination as in chapter 1.

Examination of the ear

Right ear: Pinna normal
Pre-and postaural region normal.

External auditory canal shows whitish flakes in the floor and posterior wall of the external canal.

Tympanic membrane: Color is normal, cone of light is distorted.

Handle of malleus seen. Shadow of long process of incus seen. There is perforation in the attic region involving the centre and posterior part with granulation tissue seen near the posterior margin of the perforation.

Scutum appears to be eroded. Ossicles not seen through the attic perforation. Whitish flakes are seen in the attic perforation which is difficult to remove by dry mopping.

Left ear normal.

Tuning fork test:

	Right	*Left*
Rinne	Negative	Positive
Weber	Lateralized to the left	
ABC	Reduced	Same as examiner

Patient appears to have mixed hearing loss in the right ear.

What are the causes for sensorineural loss in chronic otitis media?

- Labyrinthine involvement
- Bacterial toxin entering through round membrane
- Ototoxic topical drops entering through round window membrane.

Facial nerve—normal
Fistula test—negative

No spontaneous nystagmus
No gaze induced nystagmus
Untenberger test-negative

Romberg's sign—patient does not fall to any side with eyes open or close.
Nose—normal
Throat

Diagnosis: Chronic otitis media squamosal type active with mixed hearing loss right ear with no complications.

What are the types of chronic otitis media squamous type?

- *Inactive type*—retraction pocket in attic/may be associated epidermidiasation (i.e. change of middle mucosa to squamous epithelium) without retention of debris.
  In pars tense—self cleansing retraction pocket
  Incudostapedial joint erosion
  Structures such as stapedius tendon when seen indicates erosion of bony canal wall at level of tympanic membrane
  Adherence of tympanic membrane to promontory

- *Active squamous otitis media*
  Presence of cholesteatoma with matrix and if infected a malodorous smell. A small crust of wax in the attic may actually hide a cholesteatoma behind it. There may be erosion of ossicular chain but cholesteatoma may bridge the gap between the ossicles and so hearing loss may not be significant. Active inflammation of mucosal and submucosal region of middle ear cleft may result in polyps. Bone resorption and osteitis may manifest as granulation tissue.

How does cholesteatoma destroy bone?

Liposaccharides which are found in the cell wall of bacteria convert preosteoclastic cells to osteoclasts provided the preosteoclastic cells have been primed by receptor activator NF-KB (RANKL).

The preosteoclastic cells release cytokinase to perpetuate bone destruction. Nitric oxide is formed by cytokines, 1L10 and TNF-∞ and 1 FN-g which enhances osteoclastic activity. Proliferative factor K1-67 is elevated in cholesteatoma to show that cell homoeostasis and apoptosis are not maintained. Biofilms are also seen in extracellular matrix of cholesteatoma.

What are the causes of granulation in the external auditory canal?

- Tuberculous otitis media
- COM with cholesteatoma
- Skull based osteomylitis
- Wegener's granuloma
- Glomus jugulare.

What is the etiology of cholesteatoma?

If desquamated epithelium of the external canal accumulates in the temporal bone it is known as cholesteatoma.

External auditory canal cholesteatoma refers to accumulated keratin which has caused focal necrosis of part of bony canal wall.

Congenital: seen as white mass behind drum, with no history of otitis media and normal tympanic membrane. It can originate from vestigial structures resulting in epidermoid formation seen in the anterior tympanum resulting in an epidermal cyst. It can also be due to invagination of epidermis from developing external auditory canal or from swallowing of epidermal tissue in amniotic fluid.

It may present as late as the fourth or fifth decade of life.

Acquired cholesteatoma may be due to:

- *Invagination:* Invagnation as in retraction pocket, deepening, mouth narrowing and forming a non-cleansing cyst
- *Metaplasia:* Middle ear mucosa if exposed for long can undergo metaplasia to squamous epithelium

- *Migration:* Migration of external canal epithelium through marginal perforation
- Basal cell hyperplasia.

Iatrogenic cholesteatoma: When epithelium is left behind on handle of malleus during myringoplasty or any trauma to the tympanic membrane during surgery can cause implantation of squamous epithelium into middle ear. This is called residual cholesteatoma. Recurrent is one that occurs after surgery.

How will you investigate?

- Examination under microscope:
  - Look for site of perforation (sometimes a small crust may hide an attic perforation)
  - Look for granulations and polyps
  - Look at retraction pockets to see whether the base is seen; is it a self cleansing pocket
  - Look for cholesteatoma flakes
  - Look for ossicular destruction
  - Look for destruction of scutum/bony meatal wall
- Pure tone audiometry
- Ear swab for culture and sensitivity
- X-ray both mastoids
- CT scan—none of the indications for scan are present in this case.

How will you treat polyps associated with chronic otitis media?

It is best to remove polyps and do definitive surgery at the sametime. Polyps may be attached to ossicular chain or facial nerve.

How will you treat the patient?

Canal wall down mastoidectomy where the cholesteatoma can be followed from attic outwards (transmeatal approach) or from masoid antrum inwards (transcortical).

Transmeatal approach may result in a smaller cavity.

In transmeatal approach surgery can stop when disease stops, i.e. if only attic is involved, atticotomy or if antrum is also involved atticoantrostomy.

Indication for canal wall down mastoidectomy:

- Low lying dura/forward placed sinus causing contracted antrum and hence poor access to epitympanum
- Fistula in horizontal semicircular canal
- To get access to posterior tympanum particularly if sinus tympanic is deep
  - Rigid telescopes give good access to posterior tympanum
  - Always open facial recess in pars tensa cholesteatoma
  - Large cavity can be made small with bone pate or hydroxyl apatite granules. A vascular fascio-periosteal flap is needed to cover it.

What is facial recess and sinus tympanic?

Facial recess is a groove between pyramid and facial nerve and tympanic annulus. Its boundaries are facial nerve medially, laterally tympanic annulus and chorda tympanic nerve and superiorly the fossa incudis. Opening into the facial recess through these boundaries is known as posterior tympanotomy (widely used in cochlear implants). Extended facial recess approach involves cutting of chorda tympanic nerve to get better access to posterior tympanum. The lateral boundary of the extended facial recess approach is the annulus.

Sinus tympanic—medial wall is continuous with posterior part of medial wall of middle ear where it is related to round and oval window and subiculum of promotory. It can have aircells and can be an inaccessible area during cholesteatoma surgery. Subiculum is a bony extension of the promontory which separates the round and oval windows.

Ponticulus runs from the promontory above the subiculum and reaches the pyramid on the posterior wall. The sinus tympani lies medial to the facial nerve between subiculum and ponticulus. The round window niche is triangular and has an anterior wall, posterosuperior and posteroinferior walls. The place where the posterosuperior and posteroinferior wall meets points to the sinus tympani.

How do you approach attic through antrum?

Follow tegmen anteriorly and thin superior and posterior canal wall. Drill out zygomatic root and enter the attic. Cog is a thin flat bony projection from the tegmen. As it lies over processes cochleariformis it forms a small aperture leading to anterior attic. If this is not identified and opened disease is left behind in the anterior attic region.

What are the reasons for failure of cholesteatoma surgery?

- Posterior mesotympanum cholesteatoma
- Cholesteatoma around ossicles (now fiber guided laser can be used to remove cholesteatoma around ossicle and posterior mesotympanum.

How to get a dry ear following cholesteatoma surgery?

- Intact canal wall technique
- Do wall down only in small mastoid air cell system
- Obliterate mastoid cavity (fat/bone pate).

If canal wall down is done:

- Smooth cavity without recesses will prevent heaping and epithelialization
- Reduce facial ridge adequately (most important)
- Adequate meatoplasty (size of surgeon's thumb). A bit of conchal cartilage should be excised
- Reconstruct canal wall/bone pate or cartilage
- Remove all cells, particularly tegmen cells, sinodural angle cells, mastoid tip cells and facial recess.

What is bridge, ridge, anterior and posterior buttress?

Bridge is the bone between dura and facial ridge. Preserving the bridge either completely or partially prevents recurrent cholesteatoma.

Ridge is the bone over the facial nerve. The ridge is reduced in canal wall down surgeries.

Anterior buttress is the place where the posterior meatal wall meets the tegmen antri and removal makes the tegmen antri continuous with tegmen tympani. This is reduced in canal wall down procedures.

Posterior buttress is the bony bridge between the ear canal and the bone covering the lateral semicircular canal. This is reduced in canal wall down surgeries. Posterior buttress can also be seen as the place where the posterior canal wall meets the floor of the external auditory canal lateral to the facial nerve.

At the end of a wall down procedure the floor of the mastoid tip should be flush with floor of the external auditory canal. Anterior tympanic wall should be drilled down to become continuous with the anterior meatal wall.

Which is the ossicle most likely to be destroyed and how will you do ossiculoplasty?

- Lenticular process of incus is likely to be destroyed most frequently
- Patients own incus can be modified to bridge the gap between malleus and stapes. The autologous graft undergoes creeping substitution where nonviable bone is replaced by viable bone
- Cortical bone can also be used
- Cartilage develops chondromalacia and is hence not a good material to use
- Synthetic material such as PORP and TORP (partial ossicular chain replacement prosthesis and total ossicular chain replacement prosthesis) result in foreign body reaction with micro degradation of prosthesis
- Bio active glass (hydroxylapatite, titanium, gold, bioglass, ceravital) can also be used. Prosthesis should have low mass/low stiffness

What are the factors for failed ossiculoplasty?

- Non-aeration of middle ear cavity
- Formation of adhesion.

Describe outcomes after ossiculoplasty

- Eighty percent have airbone gap of 0–20 dB
- Ten percent have airbone gap of up to 50 dB
- Nature of prosthesis does not influence closure of gap
- If stapes superstructure is not present results are not good
- If incus alone is lost 68% success
  If incus and stapes are lost 46% success
- If malleus and stapes super structure is present results are good
  Results are worse after 5 year follow-up
- If only stapes super structure is present, less effective
- In adhesive otitis/tympanosclerosis readhesion occurs.

Long-term results of ossicular reconstruction:
- Late failure may be due to adhesion or new bone formation
- Cochlea function should be good
- Eustachian tube should function. Preoperative testing of eustachian tube function does not ensure that it will function well postoperatively.

What is Belfast rule of thumb?

To evaluate hearing in an operated ear/postoperative hearing will be useful to patient if:
- Air conduction threshold is less than 30 dB
- The air conduction threshold is within 15 dB of the air conduction threshold in the better contralateral ear. This is most important because air-bone gap should not be more than 50 dB.

How will you treat retraction pockets?

- Leave it alone surgical management of self cleaning cavity not needed
- Can be excised and grafted
- Reinforcement graft such as cartilage and fascia can be used. Tragal or conchal cartilage can be used. Palisading or thin sheets of cartilage can be prepared and placed between two temporalis fascia grafts. Tissue glue can be used to maintain position
  This is not a definitive cure as recurrence is possible
- Retracted umbo may require malleolar head excision and stapes to malleus assembly. Amputation of umbo may reduce acoustic transmission and hence better not done.

What is the effect of long-standing retraction?

- Collection of debris
- Flappy tympanic membrane
- Erosion or loss of incus. In adults pars flaccida retraction is more likely to result in cholesteatoma where as in children pars tensa retraction can cause cholesteatoma.

What is the cause of sensorineural loss after mastoidectomy?

- Effect of drill
- Ossicular chain trauma
- Blood entering labyrinth
- Infection: 2% develop dead labyrinth after mastoidectomy.

What are the indications for radical mastoidectomy?

- Eustachian tube and petrous apex cholesteatoma
- Promontory/cochlear fistula
- Chronic perilabyrinthine osteitis
- Neoplasia of temporal bone.

Chapter
3

Facial Nerve Palsy

A 40-year-old agriculturist presents in the outpatient with inability to close his right eye completely since 3 days.

HISTORY OF PRESENT ILLNESS

Patient says he was alright 3 days ago when he developed this problem. He also notices that people at home say his smile is one sided and he finds it difficult to retain food in the mouth on the right side.

Patient has no history of trauma. Patient gives history of scanty ear discharge right side which does not bother him. He has had this for a long time (3–5 years) and as it does not create any problem. He did not see a specialist. He has occasionally used ear drops. There is no foul smell or blood staining of discharge.

- No loss of taste
- No tearing of eyes
- No hard of hearing/no phonophobia (irritation of stapedius tendon)
- No vertigo/tinnitus.

Ask all other history for ear disease as in chapter 1.
No history of fever/night sweats/loss of appetite/weight loss/cough *(tuberculous otitis media can present with facial palsy).*

GENERAL EXAMINATION

Examination of face

Tests for facial nerve function

- Wrinkling of forehead absent on right side *(frontal head of occiptofrontalis)*
- Eye closure: incomplete on right side *(orbicularis oculi)*
- Inability to puff cheek right side *(buccinator)*
- Clenching of teeth causes deviation of angle of mouth to right *(orbicularis oris)*
- In upper motor neuron lesion the top half of the face is spared, i.e. wrinkling of forehead is not lost. So this is a lower motor neurone paralysis of right facial nerve.

Examination of ears

Right ear: pinna, pre and postauricular region normal, external auditory canal shows whitish debris on the floor

Tympanic membrane: posterior superior region of pars tensa there are granulations and retraction is seen, no clear perforation seen

Left ear is normal.

Tuning fork test: normal hearing

Fistula test—negative

All vestibular tests normal

Diagnosis: right facial nerve palsy (lower motor neurone) secondary to chronic otitis media squamosal type right ear (active).

How will you proceed?

1. Examination of ear under microscope.
2. Ear swab for culture and sensitivity.
3. PTA/tympanometry for acoustic reflex.
4. X-ray both mastoids.

What are topo diagnostic tests?

1. Schirmer's test: strips of blotting paper is placed on the lower fornix of each eye and length of wetness compared after 5 minutes.
   If lesion is above greater superficial petrosal nerve than there will be less tearing on involved side.
2. Stapedial reflex: if lesion is above stapedius tendon reflex is absent.
3. Electrogustometry: if lesion is above chorda tympani nerve taste is lost
4. Salivary flow test: Cannulate Warthon's duct to evaluate salivary flow following stimulation with citric acid.

What are electrophysiological tests?

1. Nerve excitability test: Tests stimulation required to produce minimal muscle contraction and compare both sides. Less than 3.5 mA difference is significant and indicates poor recovery. Can be done only after 72 hours after injury.
2. Maximal stimulation test: 5 mA current is used to test muscle contraction on both sides. Results can be equal, reduced, or absent. If loss of response occurs within 10 days it is associated with incomplete recovery.
3. Electroneuronography: stimulate nerve at stylomastoid foramen and measure biphasic myopotentials of muscles with surface electrodes. Better than 1 and 2 tests as it is a quantitative measure. It is of value after 3 days (after Wallerian degeneration has set it) but not after 3 weeks.
   If there is less than >90% response after 14 days it has poor prognosis in Bell's palsy.
   If there is less than >90% after 6 days following trauma, surgical intervention is needed.

4. *Electromyography*—useful after 2 weeks:
   a. If active motor potentials are present on voluntary action than prognosis is good
   b. If there is defibrillation potential than Wallerian degeneration has set in polyphasic myopotentials suggest reinnervation.

What is the role of HRCT?

HRCT is good in temporal bone trauma. Take axial and coronal views.

In coronal images facial nerve is the medial of the two circular eyes above cochlea. Locate pyramid/facial nerve is just behind.

B-line: A tangential line drawn from posterior border of basal turn of cochlea. This falls within 1 mm of facial nerve.

What are the causes of recurrent facial nerve paralysis?

1. Idiopathic (Bell's palsy).
2. Melkerson Rosenthal syndrome.
3. Tumor of VII N ipsilateral recurrence seen in malignant tumors contralateral recurrence is seen in benign tumors.
4. Herpes simplex-type I.

What is the cause of alternating facial nerve palsy?

Melkersson-Rosenthal syndrome.

What are the causes of bilateral concurrent facial palsy?

1. Guillian-Barre's syndrome.
2. Leukemia.
3. Sarcoidosis.
4. Lyme's disease.
5. Rabies.
6. Infections mononucleosis.
7. Mobius syndrome.

What are the degrees of facial nerve paralysis?

First degree: neuropraxia complete recovery
Second degree: axon is injured; axonotmesis/good chance of recovery, will take longer.
Third degree: disruption of neural architecture and Wallerian degeneration
Fourth and Fifth degree: partial or complete transaction of nerve
Sixth degree: epineurium is also transected.

What is House Brackman's Classification?

Salient features:
Grade I normal
Grade VI complete paralysis

Grade II and III complete eye closure
Grade IV and V eye closure incomplete
Grade V shows barely perceptible movement.

Degrees of Facial Paralysis and Brackmann's Grade Correlate

Forehead

In Grade III: Patient may not be able to lift eyebrows (corresponds to third degree/disruption of neural architecture)
In Grade IV: Inability to lift eyebrow (corresponds to fourth or fifth degree/ partial or complete transaction of nerve).

Eye

In Grade I to III: Eye closure is complete (third degree)
In Grade IV and V: Eye closure is incomplete (fourth and fifth degree).

Mouth

In Grade II: There is slight asymmetry (second degree/axon injury)
In Grade III and IV: Asymmetry of mouth (fourth degree nerve injury).

Synkinesis

In Grade II: Barely seen (only axon injury)
In Grade III: It is obvious (disruption of neural architecture)
In Grade IV: It is severe (partial tansection)
In Grade V and VI: It is absent (complete transaction).

Effort used to do these functions such as maximal effort, etc. varies from examiner to examiner.
Synkinesis: simultaneous movements of different groups as axon's branch into one another.

How will you manage traumatic facial nerve palsy following surgery?

One percent develop palsy after mastoidectomy.

When patient is recovering from anesthesia, look for movement of ala nasi.

If palsy is seen on the table, reopen, if injury is partial, persevere intact portion and repair rest.

If subtotal transection has occurred, then decompress nerve and repair if there is enough tissue.

If complete transection has occurred, then graft with greater auricular/ sural nerve.

If palsy is seen and it is within 4 hours after surgery:

- It may be due to local anesthesia but if it persists after 4 hours reopen and trace nerve from geniculate ganglion to stylomastoid foramen
- Most common part of nerve to be injured is second genu. Granulations over nerve should be removed but nerve sheath should not be opened.

In facial nerve palsy due to viral causes start famciclovir as it is better than acyclovir in crossing the blood brain barrier. Neurosurgical procedures can cause viral reactivation.

What is the cause of facial paralysis following mastoidectomy?

1. Heat of the drill.
2. Dehiscence of facial nerve canal.
3. Spicule of bone being driven into nerve.
4. Pressure of pack on exposed nerve.
5. Hematoma over nerve.
6. Transection of nerve.
7. Exerting traction on granulations over facial nerve.

What are the most common intratemporal complications of COM?

Post aural abscess—75%
Bezold abscess—2%
Facial nerve palsy—6%
Petrositis—1%
Labyrinthitis—16%

What are the most common intracranial complications of COM?

Brain abscess—25%
Subdural abscess—15%
Extradural abscess—10%
Lateral sinus thromboplebitits—20%
Meningitis—30%
Meningitis is the most common intracranial complications of COM. But, more than one complication is generally seen at the sametime.

What are routes of spread of infection?

1. Direct bony erosion.
2. Infected thrombus.
3. Emissary veins.
4. Fracture and surgical trauma (preformed pathway).
5. Normal anatomic fenestra oval window, round window, internal acoustic meatus, cochlear aqueduct.

How does a fistula occur?

Local inflammatory reaction causes osteitis and osteoclastic and osteoblastic activity. Osteoclastic activity predominant and hence leads to fistula. If inflammatory process is eliminated fistula can heal.

Fistula's can be small which is less than 2 mm in diameter and it is not likely to have involved endosteum. So it can be dissected and covered with perichondrium and fascia.

If fistula is more than 2 mm it is large, then a canal wall down mastoidectomy has to be done and close fistula at later stage (leave matrix over fistula).

Describe tuberculosis otitis media

1. Painless otorrhea.
2. Profound deafness conductive or sensorineural loss.
3. Dizziness.
4. Watery ear discharge.
5. Multiple perforation.
6. Pale middle ear mucosa.
7. Profuse pale granulation.
8. Facial nerve paralysis.
9. All cases of otitis media not responding to treatment and causing deafness disproportionate to signs suspect tuberculosis otitis media.

Describe salient features of intracranial complications

a. Meningitis: history of severe headache and pyrexia in a discharging ear. Patient is irritable. Lumbar puncture shows reduced sugar, organisms can be grown neutrophils are raised. In tuberculosis lymphocytes are raised.
b. Extradural abscess: headache may be the only symptom. Low grade pyrexia may be present.
c. Subdural abscess fits/focal neurological signs.
d. Brain abscess:
   - Temporal
   - Cerebellar.

   Signs and symptoms depend on stage of abscess. Headache/vomiting/pyrexia are the usual symptoms.
   1. Stage of cerebral edema (encephalitis signs and symptoms)
   2. Stage of inflammation
   3. Stage of walled abscess (signs and symptoms of space occupying lesion
e. Lateral sinus thrombosis: The pathology starts with phlebitis, as depicted below.

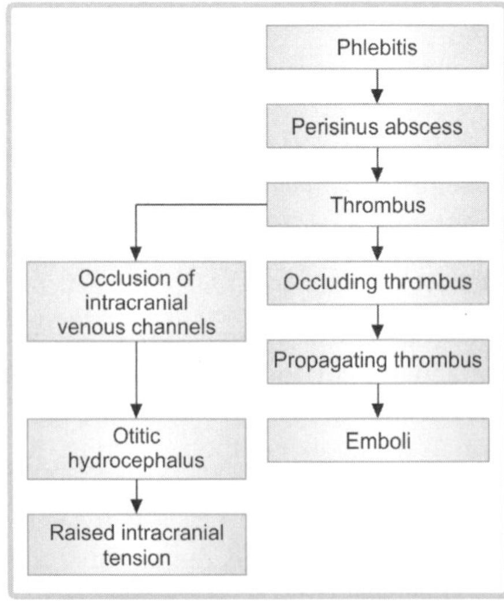

Typical fever of lateral sinus thrombus is picket fever type of fever but it may be modified by antibiotics.

If a thrombus is present, sinus plate is opened during mastoidectomy. If thrombus is soft and infected, the lateral sinus can be occluded by inserting gauze between sinus and sinus plate both above and below thrombus and then sinus is opened and thrombus evacuated.

Chapter 4

Vertigo

A 50-year-old man presents with vertigo on and off–3 weeks
(All history to be taken for vertigo as in chapter 1)

HISTORY OF PRESENT ILLNESS

How long does it last?

It lasts only for a minute or so and occurs only in some positions of the head, i.e. when I turn towards the right.

Do you feel the room is rotating or you are rotating?

The room is rotating.

Is it associated with deafness?

No

Is there ear discharge or any other ear symptoms

No

Is it episodic?

No

Is there syncope or history of migraine?

No

Are you on any long-term drugs?

No; from the history it appears to be positional vertigo.

General Examination

- ENT examination
- No abnormality seen
- Examination of vestibular system

- No spontaneous nystagmus
- No gaze induced nystagmus.

It is essential to distinguish if vertigo is of peripheral or central origin. Clinically to test visual occulomotor system.

1. Smooth pursuit.
2. Saccades.
3. Optokinetic nystagmus.
4. Vestibulo-oculomotor reflex.
5. Vestibulo-oculomotor reflex suppression.

Ocular signs indicate vestibular disorder. Central nervous system also results in eye movement which are not vestibular mediated.

If nystagmus occurs only when one eye is covered, it is called latent nystagmus and is seen in congenital occulomotor disorder.

Smooth pursuit: If target moves at reasonable speed eye follows it smoothly.
Saccades: If target moves faster than extra movements of the eye ball is needed to keep the object on the fovea. These rapid movements are called saccades.
Optokinetic nystagmus: When we look at objects from the window of a moving vehicle the eye follows the object for sometime and it is set back to central position by a fast movement. The slow ipsidirectional and fast contra directional eye movements constitute optokinetic nystagmus.
In all the 3 previous reflexes head is steady.
Vestibulo-ocular reflex: Brain uses the information given by the vestibular system to stabilize vision on the retina. This reflex helps us to focus objects on our fovea when we are in motion. It has a slow phase movement equal in velocity to head movement but opposite in direction to head movement. The neural arc for this is scarpa's ganglion/vestibular neurone and III cranial nerve.
Vestibulo-ocular reflex suppression. The human brain can suppress vestibule ocular reflex. If there is abnormality in suppressing vestibulo-ocular reflex, then there is a central lesion.

Clinical test for 1–5

1. *For smooth pursuit:* Move finger slowly in front of patient and watch for eye pursuit. If it is smooth and not broken than lesion is peripheral. If there is jerky movement or cog wheel movement than smooth pursuit is abnormal and the lesion is central.
2. *For saccades:* Ask patient to look back and forth between the examiner's index finger's placed horizontally or vertically apart
   - Saccades are small in amplitude, low in velocity or asymmetrical
   - Abnormal saccades are a sign of central lesion.
3. *Optokinetic nystagmus:*
   - This can be tested with a small drum which has stripes in black and white. The drum is rotated slowly. If drum is not available an open book can be used and patient asked to move his eyes, slowly in one direction and than in the opposite direction. The eye follows the object slowly and is reset to the centre by a quick component

- Optokinetic nystagmus may show directional preponderance. Right may beat more than left
- In central nervous system disorders the generation of fast phase contralaterally and slow phase ipsilaterally and so directional preponderance to right may be because left saccades and right pursuit is not normal.

4. Vestibulo-ocular reflex can be tested by:
   - Doll's eye manoeuvre
   - Dynamic visual acuity
   - Head thrust test.

   An easy way to look for vestibulo-ocular reflex is to shake the index finger at arms length from left to right at increasing speed. After 1 Hz, eye cannot follow finger and the image of the finger is blurred. Now if finger is fixed and head is moved even up to 5 to 6 Hz the image is not blurred. This is effective VOR.

   Doll's eye manoeuvre: Patient sits opposite examiner and fixes gaze straight ahead and patient head is rotated from side to side at 0.5–1 Hz. This speed is too fast for smooth pursuit to act. Slow eye movements cannot keep up with the target so saccades occur to keep up with the target. This can be observed.

   Dynamic visual acuity test: Move head of patient as he is reading visual acuity chart. If patient is normal his visual acuity will not change from his baseline measurement or it may change by one line. If he is not able to read 3 lines then patient's vestibulo-ocular reflex is reduced.

   Head thrust test: Described as in chapter 1.
5. Vestibulo-ocular reflex suppression: Ask patient to clasp his hands together in front of him while putting up his thumb as a target. Then patient rotates from side to side. If there is break through nystagmus it indicates central lesion. Patients with peripheral vestibular lesion have normal vestibulo-ocular reflex suppression.

Dix Hallpike maneuver should be done for positional nystagmus (see chapter 1).

Clinically also do:
1. Untenberger's test.
2. Romberg's test.
3. Tests for cerebellar dysfunction.
4. Test for cranial nerve function.

Tests in the laboratory:
1. Electronystagmography or electrooculography.
2. Rotation tests.
3. Posturography.
4. Vestibular evoke myogenic potential test.

1. Electronystagmograph (ENG): It is good. i) It quantifies data which can be used for follow-up or legal cases; ii) It tests each ear separately.

   Disadvantages:
   a. Tests only horizontal canal.

b. Tortional movement is not recorded as movement of eye falls outside electrodes.
c. Due to fatigability of vestibular nystagmus it may be normal in benign paroxysmal positional vertigo (BPVV) or Meniere's.
d. Patient should not have vestibular sedation 4 days prior to ENG.

This uses the principle that retina is negative in relation to cornea which is positive. Skin electrodes are used one on each side of the orbit.

When eyes are straight ahead the potential is 1 mV, if eyes move, potential changes and can be recorded and measured.

Right side movement is upwards and left movement is downwards.

So the test involves looking for:

1. Spontaneous nystagmus.
2. Visually guided eye movements such as smooth pursuit, saccades, optokinetic nystagmus.
3. Calorie test/rotation test.

Nystagmus of peripheral origin is suppressed by visual fixation by Frenzel's glasses. So nystagmus of peripheral origin is enhanced in a dark room and central origin nystagmus does not change in the dark.

Nystagmus recorded has a saw toothed appearance whereas central nystagmus does not have a distinct fast phase.

Peripheral nystagmus follows Alexander's law of increasing when looking towards fast component.

Saccades, smooth pursuit can be recorded by using computer generated targets. Optokinetic nystagmus can be recorded by using a large drum with stripes.

Vestibulo-ocular reflex's usually recorded by doing calorie test or rotational test.

Calorie test: Temperature changes in external auditory canal can stimulate *vestibular system* can test one ear at a time as opposed to the rotation test.

Head is raised to 30° when patient is in supine position so that horizontal canal is vertical.

Thermal changes cause convection currents resulting in cupular deflection.

Water at 30° and 44°C are used. The usual order is:

Left cold

Right cold

Left warm

Right warm

Every irrigation lasts 40 seconds. A gap of 5 minutes should exist between two irrigations.

The direction of nystagmus is cold opposite/warm same side. COWS (cold opposite warm same) or ACTH (away cold towards hot).

Measurement are taken of the velocity of the slow phase component.

The finding can be:

1. Canal paresis.
2. Directional preponderance.

3. Abnormal VOR suppression. After normal response of 80–160 seconds (following each irrigation) is over if eye is seen without fixation than nystagmus will extend by 20–60 seconds. A value less than 20 seconds indicates loss of VOR suppression and indicates a central lesion.
4. In posterior fossa disease, nystagmus occurs in plane other than expected (horizontal). This is called perverted nystagmus.

Rotation tests:
1. If both labyrinths are involved it can define extent of disease.
2. It can test abnormalities in vestibulo-ocular system.
   The test can be; sinusoidal or velocity step test (rotation in a chair).

Sinusoidal test: Patient's velocity is sinusoidally modulated and eye velocity is recorded.
Three results are possible:
1. Bilateral reduction or loss of response as seen in ototoxicity, etc.
2. Directional preponderance or asymmetric response
3. Vestibulo-ocular reflex loss shows central lesion.

Velocity step test: Patient can also be rotated in a chair with increasing velocity. Nystagmus is maximal immediately after acceleration or deceleration and then it decays.

Examination of Postural Balance

Posture: In vestibular involvement, there is a head tilt to the involved side. Romberg's test is usually positive only in acute vestibular failure.
Walking in a straight line with eyes closes may make patient fall towards side of lesion in vestibular failure.

In posturography patient is tested first with eyes open and then he is tested with eyes closed and platform stable. So the test system has platform and a visual surround.
Test is conducted with:
1. Eyes open/platform stable/normal.
2. Eyes closed/platform stable/dependence on proprioception and vestibular system.
3. Eyes open/platform stable/visual imaging distorted and this reaches balance controlling mechanism. Brain has to disregard this and depend on vestibular and proprioceptive mechanism.
4. Eyes open/platform sway/dependence on vestibular and ocular system.
5. Eyes close/platform sway/dependence only on vestibular system.
6. Eyes open/distorted imagery/platform sway/dependence on vestibular system.

Posturography helps in rehabilitation.

A inexpensive way to do the test is foam and dome test. Instead of sway platform, rubber foam is used and visual imaging can be altered using a Chinese lamp. This is of value in vestibular testing for people with congenital nystagmus.

How will you test vestibular functions in a person with congenital nystagmus?

By asking the question whether caloric induced symptoms are same as those experienced by the patient. This gives support to the fact that it is peripheral nystagmus.

What the tests for saccular functions?

That we are vertical is not managed only by otolith organ alone, but also by cues from ocular and proprioceptive mechanism.

Subjective visual vertical test can be done. Here patient sits opposite a straight luminous line. The patient should set the line in what he thinks is vertical. The line can be remote controlled. In normal patients line is set to 1–2° of real vertical.

It can be skewed to 8–10° indicates not just otolith function abnormality but abnormality of vestibular system and brain stem due to imbalance in tortional ocular system.

What is click evoked vestibular myogenic potential?

Saccule is activated with sound and changes in spinovestibular reflex. This is calculated by measuring muscular activity in the neck using eletromyogram. Patients with saccular disease such as Meniere's disease have reduced response, whereas superior semicircular canal dehiscence shows larger than normal response.

Intense sound can evoke vestibular response through stimulation of inferior vestibular nerve. Electromyogram tests the relaxation of ipsilateral sternomastoid muscle. This test is useful for superior semicircular canal dehiscence because test can be elicited even with low threshold sound and the response to the stimulus is elevated.

What are the features of superior semicircular canal dehiscence?

1. Tullio phenomenon (loud sound produces nystagmus)
2. Pressure over tragus causes nystagmus.
3. Hennebert's sign is positive.
4. Valsalva also induces nystagmus.
5. Ossiculopsia in response to loud noise.

What the differences between Peripheral and Central Vertigo?

True vertigo room turns and surroundings rotate	Patient does not experience rotation of surrounding
Associated ear problem like ear discharge hard of hearing tinnitus	No associated ear symptoms
Syncope not likely	Syncope is transient, black outs may be presents

Cont...

Cont...

Vertigo of peripheral origin usually does not last longer than 3 weeks as compensation occurs	Can last for long
Examination may reveal ear pathology	No ear pathology
Nystagmus has a distinct slow and fast component Has a latent period and is fatigable. Mostly horizontal nystagmus follows Alexander's law	No slow and fast component, no latent period and not fatigable. May be pendular/sinusoidal can be any plane. Gaze paretic nystagmus when eye is eccentric it is brought back by a slow phase nystagmus and saccades take it back to eccentric position. There is difficulty in holding eccentric gaze
Gait test: walking with eye closed in a straight line may cause unsteadiness and reveal unsuspected bilateral vestibular failure. In unilateral lesions, patient falls towards hypoactive labyrinth	In central lesion/spinal cord lesions there may be problem in step initiation and broad based gait
Normal smooth pursuit, saccades and optokinetic nystagmus rules out central cause	Abnormal smooth pursuit, saccades and optokinetic nystagmus is seen in central lesions
Vestibulo-ocular reflex suppression is normal or supranormal	Vestibulo-occular reflex suppression is lost

How is Alexander's law explained?

In unilateral acute vestibular loss the neural integration does not work and eye tends to drift to the original position. This is called leaky integer. There is an addition of this to the slow phase nystagmus which result from unilateral loss. ASo if left labyrinth is involved.

If patient looks ahead no integer is in action

R L

Slow phase to left and fast phase to right.

If patient looks to the right then leaky integer tries to bring it to center. This drift is in addition to slow phase of nystagmus so slow phase velocity increase and naturally nystagmus appeared to be exaggerated.

If patient looks towards the slow phase (that is to left) eyes tries to come to center, so slow phase velocity is reduced.

What is ossiculopsia?

There is a perception of movement of surrounding. If it is happens during head movement vestibulo-ocular reflex is not normal, if it happens in some positions it is central positional vertigo. If it is not related to movement of head it is probably central in origin. Ossiculopsia is seen in superior semicircular canal dehiscence as a response to loud noise.

Treatment of vertigo: Depends on the cause. It usually involves vestibular rehabilitation exercises, vestibular sedatives and repositioning maneuvers.

Chapter 5

Hard of Hearing

What are the investigations for a patient presenting with hearing loss?

1. Pure tone audiometry (described in chapter 1)
2. Tympanometry.

In a mechanical system the ease with which energy will flow through the system is admittance and the resistance it offers is impedance. Together it is called immittance. In the ear it is tested by a probe tone of 226 HZ delivered at 85 dBSPL. The sound pressure level is measured by an immittance meter and any change is noted as the change in energy flowing through the system.

Three measurements are made:

1. Tympanometry
2. Static immittance
3. Acoustic threshold limits
   1. In *tympanomety*, the pressure in the external auditory canal is varied and the acoustic immittance studied. In normal ears maximum transmission occurs at atmospheric pressure.
      - Type A tympanogram has its maximum peak at Organization of Department and Program Advisors (ODaPA)
      - If there is fluid in the middle ear it is flat and called type B
      - In Eustachian tube dysfunction there is retracted drum due to loss of middle ear pressure. So the peak of the tympanogram is in the negative. This means maximum transmission of sound occurs when external canal pressure is negative and this is "C" type tympanogram
      - If ossicular chain is fixed than a shallow. As type tympanogram is seen where *s* stands for stiffness
      - If ossicular chain is unduly mobile as in thin tympanic membrane or ossicular chain discontinuity then energy flow is enhanced and it is called Ad. 'd' denotes discontinuity
      - In children 1000 Hz probe tone demonstrated fluid in the middle ear which may be normal with 226 Hz probe.

2. Static immittance measures only middle ear contribution; it compares the peak at ODaPA with immittance when the air pressure is +200 daPa: Values below 0.3 cc or above 1.6 cc are evidence of middle ear disorder. Because range is so wide, some mild middle ear disorders can be missed. If immittance is 0.2 cc than there is stiffness of middle ear mechanism.
3. Avoustic reflex threshold: If sound is presented to the ear stapedius muscle of both ears contract to increase impedance. If sound is applied to right ear. Ipsilateral right/uncrossed and contralateral left/crossed occurs. If sound is applied to left ear; contralateral right/crossed & ipsilateral left/uncrossed occurs.

   Sound is presented at 85 dB at 500 to 4000 Hz frequency

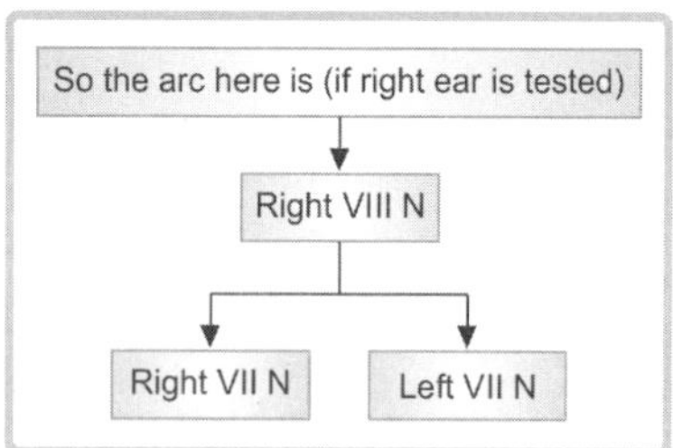

So sound traveling along right VIII N causes an ipsilateral/uncrossed VII N response and a contralateral/crossed VII N response.

SPAR: is based on difference between acoustic reflex threshold for pure tone and broadband noise. Threshold to broadband noise is lower than pure tones signals. But in sensorineural loss threshold to broadband noise is higher than for pure tone.

Threshold measurement can also be used to distinguish between cochlear and retrocochlear loss. Reflex threshold occurs at reduced sensation level in cochlear loss and they are elevated or absent in retrocochlear lesion.

If tympanic membrane is perforated increase pressure is external canal until there is a sudden fall due to opening of eustachian tube. In healthy ears slight positive pressure remains. This test can also be done when patient is swallowing.

What are the Eustachian tube functions?

Tests for eustachain tube functions:

1. Tests that measure passage of air.
2. Tests that measures opening of tube.
   a. Valsalva: pinch nose and exhale with mouth cross.
   b. Toynbee: swallow with mouth closed.
   c. Step inflation/deflation tympanometry test: In cases of intact or perforated tympanic membrane, tympanometry can be done for testing function of eustachian tube. A negative and positive pressure –200 or +200 mm of water is created while patient is asked to swallow 5 times in 20 seconds. The ability to equilibrate the pressure suggests normal Eustachian tube function.

d. Sonometry: It measures sound of opening of eustachain tube. Sound is applied in the nose and a microphone in the ear picks up the sound. SPL of 5 dB or more in the external canal indicates tubal opening.

What are the functions of Eustachain tube?

1. Pressure equalization.
2. Mucociliary clearance and drainage.
3. Middle ear protection.
4. Sound protection.

Describe the anatomy of Eustachain tube

It has bony 1/3 and cartilaginous 2/3. The opening in mesotympanum is oval to triangular and not dependent.

The bony part is related to temperomandibular joint laterally and inferiorly and middle cranial fossa superiorly, internal carotid artery is medial. In pneumatised mastoid 33% have peritubal cells.

The cartilaginous part has a large medial lamina and smaller lateral lamina. It is fixed in a groove in the greater wing of sphenoid. Nasopharyngeal end lies opposite posterior end of inferior turbinate.

Dilator of eustachain tube is tensor veli palatini muscle.

The fossa of Rosenmüller is related to petrous apex.

3. Otoacoustic emission is a test of outer hair cell functions
   - Spontaneous otoacoustic emissions occur without any sound stimulus. It is absent in ears with sensorineural loss above 30 dB. It is absent in 50% of normal ears. A microphone in the external canal measures this sound as it is absent in 50% of normal ears it cannot be used as a test
   - Evoked otoacoustic emissions have to be used. It is of two types, transient evoked otoacoustic emissions and distortion product otoacoustic emission
   - Transient evoke otoacoustic emission occur as a response to click signal at 80-85 dB. The responses are analyzed on a graph depicting amplitude versus frequency. If magnitude of emissions exceeds magnitude of signal and if reproducibility of emission exceeds predetermined level then emission is present and it is normal
   - In distortion product otoacoustic emission two tones are presented designated f1 and f2 and so distortion occurs. The best distortion is seen in the frequency 2 f1–f2. Tones are used from 1,000–6,000 HZ .This is plotted on a graph with frequency on x axis and amplitude in dB on y-axis. Emission should exceed normal background noise to be considered normal and it means outer hair cells are functioning well for f2 frequency
   - Otoacoustic emission is a good screening test for detecting hearing loss in children. It is used as a screening test in all countries for their universal hearing screening program.

4. Auditory evoke potential
   - In response to sound, portions of the auditory system generates a waveform called auditory evoke potential
   - The waveform which occurs within 5 milliseconds of presentation of sound is electrocochleogram. This tests cochlea and proximal VIII nerve. Electrocochleogram has 3 responses: Summation potential, action potential and cochlear microphonics
   - Cochlear microphonics mimics stimulus
   - Action potential is response by nerve fibers
   - Summation potential precedes action potential
   - The important measurements are action potential latency, amplitude between SP and action potential
   - This is not an ideal test, as the probe has to be close to the promontory
   - The response which occurs within 10 milliseconds is auditory brainstem evoke response (ABR). This is the response from distal VIII N to mid brain
   - 50 millseconds MLR (middle latency reflex). This is the response from auditory cortex
   - 250 milliseconds the response is LLR or (late latency reflex). This is the response from primary auditory cortex and associated areas of cerebral cortex
   - These are all evoked by a single stimulus and have a transient nature
   - ASSR is auditory steady state potential and is recorded by modulating change in stimulus. Response to slower rate comes from central part of the system, while response to faster rate comes from peripheral system
   - Auditory brain stem evoke response (ABR) has 5 positive peaks.

   Wave I: distal end of VIII N 2 milliseconds

   Wave II: proximal portion of nerve near brain stem

   Wave III: proximal portion of nerve near brain stem and cochlear nucleus. 4 milliseconds.

   Wave IV and V: cochlear nucleus, superior olivary body, and lateral lemniscus. The inter peak latency from Wave I to Wave V is about 4 milliseconds.

   ABR:

   1. Can be recorded by surface electrodes.
   2. Response is not influenced by patient's condition such as sleep/sedation.
   3. Waves are uniformly produced and is constant across people.
   4. Interpeak intervals are prolonged in retrocochlear loss and so can be used to differentiate between cochlear and retrocochlear loss.
   5. To detect small tumors of VIII N, instead of using only high frequency range as is done normally, a broadband frequency is used and summated wave V results are used to detect small tumors. This is stacked ABR.
   6. Each laboratory has its own normative data.

MLR: It can be used to detect problems such as auditory processing disorder. It has two positive peaks.

LLR: It has a negative and positive peak but it is not well developed in infancy and childhood, and is best seen only in the awake state. Abnormality or absence denotes auditory processing disorder.

What happens to ABR in conductive hearing loss?

A 30 db conductive hearing loss causes 90 db ABR waveform to resemble one elicited at 60 db in a normal ear. Absolute latencies are delayed but interwave latencies are not affected. Otoacoustic emission is absent in conductive hearing loss, if the loss prevents sound from reaching cochlea.

When is ABR considered abnormal?

ABR is abnormal if:

1. There is an interaural latency difference in I-V interpeak interval.
2. I-V interpeak interval.
3. Interaural difference in wave V frequency latency.
4. Absolute latency of wave V.
5. Interaural difference in V/I amplitude ratio.
6. Wave V/I amplitude ratio.
7. Selective loss of late waves.
8. Grossly degraded waveform morphology.
9. Cochlear hearing loss gives rise to acoustic reflex at reduced intensity. OAE is absent in cochlear hearing loss.

How is bone conduction perceived?

Sound travels by three routes to the cochlea

1. Skull bones to cochlea.
2. Skull bones → middle ear ossicles → cochlea.
3. Skull bones → external auditory canal → middle ear → cochlea

What is Carhart's notch?

In conductive hearing loss the 2 components of bone conduction hearing is missing, i.e. middle ear component and external auditory canal component. So there is a dip at 2 KHz in the audiogram in bone conduction. It was first seen in otosclerosis. It can occur in any conductive hearing loss.

What are the usual frequencies used to study air bone gap?

0.5, 1, 2 and sometimes 4 KHz. 10 dB gap is considered as loss. In otosclerosis, operate between 15-20 dB loss.

What is Carhart's effect?

The bone conduction curve improves by an average of 12 db over 0.5, 1 and 2 KHz after stapedectomy. This happens because, postoperative bone conduction curve appears to have improved in comparison to preoperative bone conduction curve, as external canal and middle ear factors have improved.

What is overclosure?

When postoperative air conduction curve is tested with preoperative bone conduction curve, it appears to be better than bone conduction and is called overclosure. Overclosure is seen in otosclerosis surgery and not in other surgeries for conductive hearing loss because, other surgeries do not correct hearing impairment as well as stapedectomy does.

What are the contraindications for stapedectomy?

1. Associated Meneire's.
2. In unilateral otosclerosis, benefit is perceived only if hearing improves to match normal ear. The airbone gap has to close to 10 dB.
3. Refixed stapes.
4. Only hearing ear.

What are non-surgical methods of relieving deafness?

- Hearing aid: Its components are microphone, amplifier and receiver. Microphones may be directional—a microphone converts acoustic energy to electrical energy.
  Amplifier may be digital.
- Implantable aids:
  a. Implanted to ossicles
  b. Implanted to skull bone → bone anchored hearing aid.

What is Glasgow hearing aid benefit profile?

Glasgow hearing aid benefit profile is a preferred questionnaire to assess hearing aid benefit because, it measures all three parameters such as benefit, use, and satisfaction.

- It contains both standard and individualized measures to assess benefit
- It assesses direct benefit
- It also compares disability before and after rehabilitation.

Why are implant aids preferred over hearing aids?

i. Appearance
ii. Can be used in external canal occlusion
iii. Less distortion of sound
iv. Less feedback
v. Amplification is better
vi. Can be done in discharging ears.

- Cochlear implants
  a. Parts of implants:
    - Receiver/stimulator in bony recess; electrode array goes to cochlea. These form internal device
    - Microphone/microprocessor/transmitter coil form external device

- Transmitter coil is magnetically coupled to the internal device (which has a magnet).

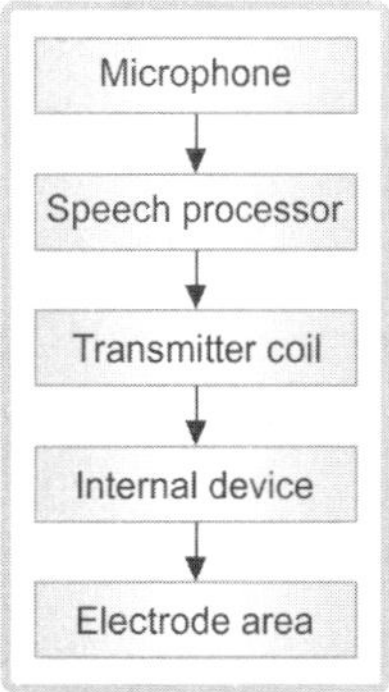

b. Types of cochlear implants generally used (name of device/country of origin):
   - Nucleus-Cochlear-Sydney Australia
   - MedEl-Innsbruck-Austria
   - Clarion-Advanced Bionic Device-California-USA
c. Conditions in which implant will work:
   - Normal cortical and central auditory system
   - Viable spiral ganglion cells and VIII N. The exact number of viable ganglion cells is not known, but at least 10% should be viable
   - Best if implanted before 2 years of age
   - Longer the duration of deafness worse the outcome in post lingual adults/children
   - Can be done even when some residual hearing is present
   - Loss of neural plasticity if deafness is of long duration. So implant may not work.
d. Investigations prior to surgical implantation:
   i. High resolution CT to look for ossified cochlea.
   ii. MRI–vestibular aqueduct
   Auditory nerve
   Internal acoustic meatus to rule out shwanomma
   Cochlear dysplasia
   Size of cochlear nerve gives an indication of number of spiral ganglion cells.
e. Surgical technique:
   - Standard postaural incision
   - Cortical mastoidectomy/posterior tympanotomy
   - Scala tympani entered via cochleostomy/use facial nerve monitor
   - Bony recess to fix receiver/stimulator
   If cochlea is ossified drill over modiolus and insert into scala vestibule.

f. Complications:
   - Facial nerve palsy/stimulation of facial nerve
   - Device failure
   - Meningitis

How to do an MRI in an implantee?

1. Remove magnet surgically.
2. Scanner equipped with 1 tesla magnet allows MRI.

Chapter 6

Deviated Nasal Septum

A 25-year-old male presents with left-sided nasal block for the past five years.

HISTORY OF PRESENT ILLNESS

I. Patient started experiencing nasal block 5 years ago which was gradual in onset and started getting worse over the past 3 years. The nasal block is continuous and does not relate to change in position.
Nasal block due to allergy and infection gets worse on lying down as secretions do not drain easily and there is mucosal edema around the sinus drainage areas in the supine position. Some causes of unilateral nasal block are:
   a. *Unilateral choanal atresia*
   b. *Deviated nasal septum*
   c. *Antrochoanal polyp when it has not occluded the nasopharynx*
   d. *Benign/malignant nasal masses/rhinolith*
   e. *Foreign bodies in the nose/unilateral foul smelling nasal discharge is usually due to an old foreign body or nasal diptheria.*

II. There is a history of nasal discharge which is watery in the mornings but on occasions it is mucoid and mucopurulent. The patient says his discharge reduces on medication such as local drops and tablets. The tablets have been given as single dose tablets and occasionally he has had 3–4 capsules for 5 days.
Nasal discharge can be watery in: Allergic and non-allergic rhinitis
Cerebrospinal fluid rhinnorhea. To distinguish between the two clinically: CSF does not stiffen linen as it has no mucoid gland secretion whereas in allergies rhinitis there is mucoid secretion. Mucoid and mucopurulent discharge is seen in chronic inflammation of the nose and sinuses.
Blood stained discharge is seen in:
   1. *Malignancies of nose and paranasal sinuses*
   2. *Chronic granulomatous lesions.*

III. Epistaxis
No history of epistaxis.
   1. *Idiopathic bleeding from little area.*

2. *Nasopharyngeal angiofibroma.*
3. *Malignancies of nose/PNS/nasopharynx.*
4. *Hypertension.*
5 *Blood dyscracias.*
6. *Rhinosporidiosis.*

These are the common causes of epistaxis.

IV. Patient has no history of bouts of sneezing, itching of the medial canthus of the eyes or around the ala nasi. No history of watering of the eyes.
These are seen in allergic/non-allergic rhinitis.

V. No history of head ache or fever.
Headache is a symptom of sinonasal disease. It is also a symptom of ophthalmic and neurological diseases. Sinonasal headache has a diurnal variation usually because the sinus secretions do not drain at night. There is no dependant drainage in the supine position; and mucosal edema in the supine position hinders drainage. Sinoanasal headaches are associated with nasal symptoms. Ophthalmic headache is worse in the evening on using vision throughout the day. It is also associated with other ophthalmic symptoms. Neurological headache can be tension headache or migraine or due to other neurological problems. Migraine is preceded by visual aura and in usually one sided and may be relieved by vomiting.

VI. No history of snoring.
Nasal block can give rise to snoring and obstructive sleep apnea.

VII. No history of visual problems.
Any space occupying lesion/malignant mass can cause visual problems.

VIII. No history of unexplained falling of teeth/dentures becoming ill fitting.
This is seen in malignancies of maxilla.

IX. No history of ear pain or discharge.
Nasal/sinonasal/nasopharyngeal pathology can result in a malfunctioning of eustachian tube.

X. No history of throat pain.
Pharyngitis causing throat pain and odynophagia can result from mouth breathing.

Past history: No history of diabetes, hypertension, tuberculosis or syphilis.

Diabetes can cause fungal rhinosinusitis with unilateral nasal block.
Many antihypertensives causes nasal block.
Tuberculosis and syphilis give rise to granulomatous lesions in the nose.
Family history: Not significant.
Personal history: Not a smoker or alcoholic.
General physical examination.
Do it as in all cases: Normal in this case.

Local Examination

Examination of the nose: The osteocartilagenous framework of the nose in normal.

The main bones of the external nose are the nasal bones. The cartilaginous framework is made up of upper and lower lateral cartilages.

a. *Physiological abnormalities like a hump, a bulbous tip or a slightly wide nose can be present.*
b. *Bony cartilaginous framework may be deformed due to previous trauma.*
c. *Fistulas or cysts may be seen over the nose.*
d. *Bilateral nasal polypi can cause widening of the nasal bridge.*
e. *A large mass in the nasal cavity can causes deformity of the external nose.*
f. *Lesions which involve skin over the nose are papular lesions of sarcoidosis/ glistening skin colored or reddish-brown nodules due to lupus vulgaris.*
g. *Saddle nose deformity of the external nose is seen.*
   1. *Following nasal surgery*
   2. *Granulomatous lesions of the nose such as Hansen's disease*
   3. *Following septal hematoma or abscess.*

   Nasal vestibule is normal.
   - *There may be presence of furuncles or apple jelly nodules in the nasal vestibule*
   - *The skin lined part of the nasal cavity in the vestibule. It is examined by lifting the tip of the nose with the left thumb*
   - *A caudal disclocation of the septum may also be seen in the vestibule sinonasal masses can present at the vestibule.*

   Cottle's test is normal.
   - *This shows that the obstruction is not in the nasal valve region.*

What is the nasal valve and false negative Cottle's test?

The nasal valve is the narrowest part of the nasal airway. It can be divided into external and internal nasal valves.

Boundaries of internal nasal valve medially—dorsal end of the septum.

Laterally—internal caudal end of upper lateral cartilage.

Posteriorly anterior end of inferior turbinate.

Boundaries of external nasal valve; caudal edge of lateral crus of lower lateral cartilage, alar fibrofatty tissue and medially the membranous septum.

Nasal valve area is the space between the internal nasal valve and pyriform aperture.

False negative Cottle's test is seen in:
a. Synechia preventing opening of nasal valve
b. Osteotomies following rhinoplasty may result in medializazation of ascending process of maxilla.

Anterior Rhinoscopy

- There is deviation of the nasal septum causing a vertical ridge in the region of the middle turbinate resulting in a c-shaped deviation of the nasal cartilage. There are no spurs or horizontal crests seen
- The left nasal cavity is narrowed and only a part of the inferior turbinate is seen. The mucosa appears pale gray in color

- The right nasal cavity is wider than the left, no spurs seen over the septum. The inferior turbinate is hypertrophied and the middle turbinate is seen. Mucosa is pale gray in color. No secretions seen in the nasal cavity or floor of the nose or middle meatus
- Posterior rhinoscopy did not reveal any abnormality. The posterior end of the septum is seen. Choana are normal, the eustachain tube orifice, torus tubaris, and fossa of Rosenmüller are normal, roof and posterior wall of the nasopharynx is normal
- Examination of the paranasal sinuses; no tenderness elicted over the canine fossa/adjacent to the medial canthus/or along the medial aspect of the supraorbital region
- Examination of the oral cavity
- No gingivolabial sulcus fullness, no loss of teeth, no palatal fullness
- Examination of oropharynx; no postnasal drip
- Cotton wool test: moves less at the left nares/right nares normal movement
- Cold spatula test: reduced fogging on the left-side
- Examination of ears: normal
- Examination of larynx: normal
- Examination of neck: no palpable neck nodes or swelling.

Diagnosis: Deviated nasal septum to the left with allergic rhinitis.

What are the investigations you would like to do?

Diagnostic nasal endoscopy using a 4.0 mm 30 degree scope and for children 2.7 mm 30 degree rigid scope.

The three passes are aimed at a systemic examination which will not miss any area.

First pass in along the floor of the nose goes through the inferior meatus, look for the nasolacrimal duct opening. Advance scope to visualize nasopharynx, look for secretions and nature of sinonasal mucosa. Secretions from the anterior group of sinuses go inferior to the eustachian tube opening where as secretions from the posterior group go superior to the eustachian tube opening.

Second pass goes between the inferior and middle turbinates to visualize middle meatus, fontanella and accessory ostia. By going medial to the posterior aspect of the middle turbinate and rotating the scope superiorly the superior turbinate and sphenoid ostea is seen.

Third pass—when withdrawing scope rotate it laterally beneath the posterior aspect of the middle turbinate to see the middle meatus. Bulla ethomoidalis/hiatus semilunaris/infundibular entrance and uncinate are seen. Look for mucosal swelling, crusts and secretions.

CT scan of the nose and paranasal sinuses/X-ray paranasal sinuses Water's view to rule out rhinosinusitis.

Do you clinically feel there is rhinosinusitis?

There are no clinically sights of sinusitis such as:

a. Congested nasal mucosa
b. Pus in the middle meatus or floor of the nose
c. Post nasal drip
d. Posterior granular pharyngitis

Are there any objective tests to confirm the presence of patients symptoms?

1. Nasal obstruction visual analog scale or Likert scale
2. Peak nasal inspiration flow
3. Acoustic rhinometry
4. Rhinomanometry
5. Olfactometry
6. Photograph
7. Test for nasal allergy

1. Likert scale uses the terms such as not obstructed, mildly obstructed moderately obstructed, severely obstructed to denote amount of nasal obstruction. In the visual analog scale patient will mark a point on a line to represent nasal obstruction.
2. Peak nasal inspiration flow measures peak air flow in litres/per minute during maximal forced nasal inspiration.
   a. Pitfall is that inspiration depends on patient cooperation. Normal inspiration is not the same as maximum forced nasal inspiration. In normal inspiration there is a lower tidal volume.
   b. Does not measure transnasal pressure difference. So it is based on patients cooperation.
   c. Maximum inspiration increases turbulent flow.
   d. Respiratory comorbidity can limit inspiratory effort. But it can test nasal patency.
3. Acoustic rhinometry
   - An acoustic impulse travelling along the nasal passage measures nasal geometry. Nasal volumes are calculated from contiguous cross sectional values
   - Acoustic rhinometry consists of a sound source, wave tube, microphone, filter, amplifier, digital converter and a computer
   - A sound wave is transmitted into the nasal cavity and it is reflected back from the nasal passages. This is converted to digital impulses which can be constructed into a rhinogram
   - First notch—nasal valve area
   - Second notch—anterior part of inferior turbinate
   - Third notch—posterior part of middle turbinate
   - CT and MRI shows results of acoustic rhinometry are reliable. It is very useful to test objective improvement following surgery or steroid therapy.

4. Rhinomanometry measures transnasal pressure and airflow. From this the:
   a. Mean pressure
   b. Volume
   c. Work (pressure x flow)
   d. Resistance (pressure divided by flow).

   of each breath can be calculated and plotted on a graph with pressure differential on the X-axis and flow on the Y-axis. It produces a S-shaped graph.

   The machine consists of:
   1. Pressure transducer for postnasal pressure
   2. Pneumotachometer to measure flow
   3. Mask for measuring anterior nasal pressure and flow
   4. Computer to convert measured signals to digital signals.

   Postnasal pressure is measured in three ways:
   1. A transducer is placed in the nose not being tested. As there is no flow in that nostril, the anterior pressure is same as posterior pressure. So we can get anterior and posterior nasal pressure airflow for each nostril.
   2. Here postnasal pressure is detected by placing a pressure detector in the posterior part of the oropharynx.
   3. The third method places a pressure trasducer in the nasopharynx using a nasopharyngeal tube on the test and nontest sides.

   Numbers 2 and 3 are not tolerated well by patients. If patients own breathing is used, it is called active rhinomanometry. If air is pumped at a known rate, it is passive rhinomanometry. Passive rhinomanometry does not mimic normal physiology.
   Airflow is measured using a nozzle or a mask at the nasal outlet.

Odisoft Rhino: Nasal airflow generates a high frequency sound as turbulence increases. This can be measured. Odisoft differs from acoustic rhinometry where sound is reflected back and measured. Odisoft Rhino results correlate with patients symptoms.

What will you do after investigations?

Patient can be posted for septoplasty.

Describe septoplasty

Two types of incisions can be made on the septum. Killian's is 1 cm behind caudal end of septum. It is difficult to treat caudal dislocation with this incision. Freer's or hemitransfixation incision is 2 mm posterior to caudal end of septum.

Elevate mucoperichondrial layer. Create anterior and inferior tunnels. Separate cartilage from perpendicular plate of ethmoid and vomer. Seperating cartilage from perpendicular plate of ethmiod is called posterior chondrotomy. After this the septum is like a swinging door and access to posterior bony septum is possible.

Other than these steps, rest of the surgery such as removing parts of cartilage, cross hatching, etc. has to be individualized for each patient.

If large parts of the septum are removed, it should be reconstructed. If cartilage is removed a dorsal and caudal strut should be left behind.

Septoplasty can also be done endoscopically either by making an incision only on the deviated part and removing it or by making the same incision as before and proceed using the endoscope.

Will you remove the inferior turbinate?

Originally it was assumed that the paradoxical nasal block experienced by the patient on the non-deviated side was due to the inferior turbinate hypertrophy; but now it considered to be due to the nasal cycle.

What is nasal cycle?

This is the alternative nasal block which occurs between the nasal passages and is caused by filling of the nasal sinusoids in the inferior turbinate. It is controlled by the autonomic nervous system and the cyclic changes occur between 4-12 hours and it is a constant for every human being. Nasal cycle is modified by various factors like allergy, infections, exercise, hormones, pregnancy, fear and emotions, etc.

In a patient with deviated septum, say to the right, patient subconsciously eliminates the resistance on the right side. But whenever there is a filling of the sinusoids on the left side, he perceives it acutely and says there is obstruction on the left side. Hence, elimination of inferior turbinate surgically may not cure this.

What are the types of septal deviation?

One classification is:

1. Anterior cartilaginous
2. Combined bony and cartilaginous

Anterior cartilaginous deviation is seen with external nasal deviation and dislocation of cartilage off anterior nasal spine. It is often seen in vaginal delivery children when face and shoulders are pressed against pelvic wall which can lead to deviated nasal septum.

Combined deviation involves vomer, perpendicular plate of ethmoid and cartilage. This occurs as a part of generalized facial deformity.

Maxillary moulding theory states all forms of deviation are parts of a spectrum.

Mladina classifies nasal deviation into 7 types:

Type I: Unilateral vertical ridge in valve region

Type II: More severe than Type I and causing obstruction of nasal valve

Type III: Unilateral vertical ridge at the level of head of middle turbinate (C shaped deviation)

Type IV: Combination of Type III with Type I or II, often described as S-shaped deviation
Type V: Horizontal septal crest in contact with lateral wall
Type VI: Horizontal crest on the deviated side with prominent maxillary crest on the contralateral side
Type VII: Combination of above described deformity types.

If obstruction is in nasal valve area, how will you correct it?

The nasal valve area can be widened using a spreader graft to stent the nasal valve. Graft is placed between septal cartilage and upper lateral cartilage. External valve can be widened using a graft placed cephalic to lower lateral cartilage.

What are the types of inferior turbinate hypertrophy and how can it be treated?

Hypertrophy can be:

a. Bony
b. Soft tissue/majority due to inflammatory causes
c. Mixed.

Total or partial turbinectomy causes crusting, bleeding and even atrophic changes.

Submucous resection of soft tissue and turbinate, out fracturing are better options.

Electrocautery, submucous injection of steroids, laser resection, radio frequency turbinate resection (induces submucosal tissue destruction), cryosurgery all give temporary relief. Microdebrider can be used in submucosal reduction of turbinate size.

What is empty nose syndrome?

Following inferior turbinectomy or middle turbinectomy the patient has a feeling of nasal obstruction (paradoxical) and crusting. This inability to perceive nasal air results in hyperventilation by the patient. It is also seen that air impinging on the nerve ending of the turbinates, results in bronchodilator effect, which is missing in empty nose syndrome.

This needs to be distinguished from atrophic rhinitis where histopathological changes are seen in the mucosa and turbinates, and there is definite presence of organisms. Paradoxical obstruction can be explained by the fact that during surgery nerve endings are cut and so when air impinges on the nasal mucosa, it is not perceived by the person.

How will you treat empty nose syndrome?

Cotton wool pledgets placed over the area of the turbinates and testing whether patient's symptoms improve is a good way of judging whether surgical implants will help. Acellular dermal graft can be placed over the septum or lateral wall corresponding to the region of the inferior turbinate.

Chapter 7

Sinonasal Polyps

A 33-year-old male presents with nasal obstruction—1 year.

HISTORY OF PRESENT ILLNESS

Patient was apparently normal one year ago. He started having nasal obstruction which was insidious in onset gradually progressing in severity. It is bilateral but worse on the left side. Initially, it was intermittent by now it is present all the time. There are no aggravating or relieving factors and no diurnal variation.

Bilateral nasal block can be intermittent or continuous.
Some causes are:

- *Intermittent*
  a. *Rhinosinusitis*
  b. *Allergic rhinitis*
- *Continuous*
  a. *Turbinate hypertrophy*
  b. *Nasopharyngeal mass*
  c. *Deviated nasal septum with turbinate hypertrophied on the opposite side*
  d. *Chronic granulomatous lesions*
  e. *Choanal atresia*
  f. *Bilateral ethmoidal polypi.*

There are no other nasal symptoms (see Chapter 6 for nasal symptoms).

Past history: No previous history of nasal surgery.
(nasal surgery involving turbinates can result in empty nose syndrome causing nasal obstruction)

- No history of asthma
  Nasal obstruction due to polyps can be associated with asthma and aspirin allergy.
- No past history of diabetes mellitus, tuberculosis or syphilis.
  Tuberculosis can involve the nasal cavity as lupus vulgaris or as a reddish nodule associated with nasal discharge and pain. The nodule usually

involves the anterior part of the nasal septum which can later ulcerate, break down and result in a perforation of the septal cartilage.

In tertiary syphilis the bony septum is involved and a perforation can occur. In the secondary stage of syphilis, there is a catarrhal rhinitis. In congenital syphilis, there is nasal discharge and nasal obstruction (snuffles).

FAMILY HISTORY/PERSONAL HISTORY

General physical examination as in all cases

On Examination

- External nose appears normal
- Nasal vestibule is normal
- Anterior rhinoscopy:
    - The left cavity is filled with multiple pale smooth masses. Only a part of the vestibule is free. Anteriorly the caudal part of the septum is seen. The masses are pale have a smooth surface, not pulsatile, not sensitive to touch and does not bleed.

(Malignant masses/inverted papilloma do not have a smooth surface and they bleed on touch).

- In the right nasal cavity, there is a single pale glistening mass with a smooth surface occupying part of the nasal cavity. The septum is seen and anterior part of the inferior turbinate is also seen
- No other structure is visible. The mass is not pulsatile, insensitive to touch, soft in consistency and does not bleed
- Probe can be passed all round the swelling in the right nasal cavity but cannot be passed laterally in the left nasal cavity
- Posterior rhinoscopy—choana is free
- Rest of examination as in Chapter 6.

Diagnosis: Bilateral sinonasal polyposis.

What is your differential diagnosis?

1. Inverted papilloma.
2. Malignant lesion lurking behind the polyp.
3. In children meningocele.
4. Allergic fungal rhinosinusitis.

Why are polypi from ethmoids multiple?

Because there are number of cells in the ethmoid region.

Why does an antrochoanal polyp present posteriorly?

1. The accessory maxillary antrum ostia is posterior.
2. The cilia beats posteriorly.
3. The slope of the nose is towards the choana.

How do you differentiate a polyp from a turbinate?

- Polyps are soft/turbinate is hard
- Polyps are insensitive/turbinates are sensitive
- Polyps do not shrink with decongestants
- Enlarged turbinates reduce in size with decongestants
- Probe can be passed all around a polyp, whereas turbinate has a lateral attachment.

What is the etiology of polyps?

Nasal polyps occur in varying frequencies with a number of specific airway diseases. 80% of allergic fungal rhinosinusitis is associated with polyps. Nonallergic rhinitis is more likely to be associated with polyps than allergic rhinitis. It is also seen in non-steroidal anti-inflammatory drug (NSAID) intolerance and asthma, cystic fibrosis, Cherry Strauss syndrome and primary ciliary dyskinesia.

There is a disruption of mucosal lining and a resultant inflammatory cascade resulting in polyposis.

If a person has reduced Th-1 based immune response, then an increased Th-2 based response is seen. The response causes chronic inflammation and increased eosinophil infiltration. There is also reduced eosinophil apoptosis. Increased chemokines such as eotaxin and regulated on activation normal T expressed and secreted (RANATES) are responsible for the increased eosinophils. Proinflammatory cytokines such as tumor necrosis factor (TNF), interferon, granulocyte macrophage colony stimulating factor and ILS are a source of increased eosinophils. Stromal edema persists because of lack of lymphangiogenesis. Eosinophilis increase local vascular permeability and mucous secretion and cause further inflammatory cell influx.

How will you investigate this patient?

1. Diagnostic nasal endoscopy.
2. Nasal secretions eosinophil count.
3. Total and differential count.
4. Tests for nasal allergy.
5. CT.
6. MRI.

Why are standard radiographs not useful?

Standard X-rays do not estimate degree of chronic inflammation in the sinuses particularly ethmoid sinus. It does not show the anatomy of the osteomeatal complex.

What are the views taken during CT of nose and PNS and why?

Coronal plane CT: It approximates the surgical approach. It is the best plane for osteomeatal complex, relationship of orbits to paranasal sinuses, relationship of brain and ethmoid roof. Scanning is done from anterior wall of frontal sinus to the posterior wall of sphenoid sinus. 3 mm cuts are taken. Scan plane within 10° of perpendicular to the hard palate best for osteomeatal complex. Even when orbit is barely visible in the scan, agger nasi cell is seen and demonstrates how anteriorly it is placed.

Axial view shows sphenoid and posterior ethmoid disease/position of internal carotid artery and optic nerve.

Sagittal cuts give an idea of the frontal recess. It also allows distance measurement for passage of instruments.

What is Hounsfield unit?

Hounsfeild unit denotes tissue density on CT. Air is -1000 units and metal is ≥ +1000 units. Blood is +80, water is 0.

What is the radiological classification of sinonasal polyps?

- 0—no opacity
- 1—some opacity
- 2—total opacity.

	Right	*Left*
Maxilla	0–2	0–2
Anterior ethmoid	0–2	0–2
Posterior ethmoid	0–2	0–2
Sphenoid	0–2	0–2
Frontal	0–2	0–2
Osteomeatal complex	0–2	0–2

How do you endoscopically stage polyps?

- No polyps—0
- Restricted to middle meatus—1
- Below middle turbinate—2
- Massive polyposis—3.

What is helical scanning?

Helical/spiral scanning permits rapid scanning of large volumes of tissue. It is a combination of continuous rotational tube head motion about the patient, along with the continuous feed of the patient through the scanner. For coronal images, patient has to lie prone with neck extended and this is not comfortable. So, a multi-row detector computer tomography (MDCT)/ spiral scanner is used. This is good for patients who cannot hyper extend neck for long periods and for patients with dental restoration. It scans a volume of tissue and provides better quality images than normal scans.

Is magnetic resonance imaging (MRI) a good aid for functional endoscopic sinus surgery (FESS)?

Cortical bone and air have no mobile protons and hence do not yield MRI signal.

Why do polyps occur in the osteomeatal complex?

1. Touching mucous membrane in the osteomeatal complex results in disruption of mucosal surfaces and release of proinflammatory cytokines from epithelial cells.
2. Influence of special air flow, air current and pressure in the upper airway.
3. Nerve endings near borderline of nose and PNS is thin and may be easily damaged by cytotoxic proteins released from eosinophils. Denervation of nasal mucosa causes loss of autonomic control resulting in secretory activities of glands, increases vascular permeability and tissue edema.

In this case how will you do a polypectomy?

Endoscopically enough polyps have to be removed anteriorly and inferiorly so that middle turbinate can be visualized. Once normal structures are identified, uncinectomy and middle meatal antrostomy can be done.

Describe uncinectomy?

Zero degree endoscope passes through middle meatus and identifies uncinate. Sometimes middle turbinate may have to be rotated medially. Uncinate is crescent shaped. Anteriorly it fuses with posteromedial wall of the agger nasi cell and posteromedial wall of the nasolacrimal duct. If has a free supero-posterior edge. Posterior to the uncinate is the bulla ethmoidalis. The free edge of the uncinate sometimes adheres to the bulla or lamina papyracea, when it is called atelectatic uncinate process. The superior attachment of the uncinate is variable. It can get attached to roof of ethmoid, middle turbinate or lamina papyrace. Depending on this the frontal sinus will open directly into the middle meatus if uncinate is attached to lamina papyracea or it will drain into the infundibulum in the other 2 instances.

Make an incision between inferior 1/3 and superior 2/3 of uncinate. Incision is carried anteriorly till lacrimal bone is reached. The uncinate can be removed using sickle knife or Freer's elevator or microdebrider.

What is basal lamella?

The middle turbinate has 3 attachments, anterior in a sagital plane it attaches to skull base, middle it attaches to the lamina papyrace in a coronal plane and posteriorly it slopes to an axial plane and is attached to the posterior aspect of the lamina. The middle vertical aspect of the middle turbinate attachment forms the basal lamella and separates anterior ethmoidal cells from posterior ethmoid cells. Posterior ethmoid cells can be opened by opening the inferior and medial aspects of the vertical basal lamella.

How do you interpret a CT of the nose and paranasal sinuses?

1. Look for all the normal structures.
2. Evaluate ethmoid roof variations.
3. Evaluate position of carotid artery and optic nerve to posterior ethmoid and sphenoid.
4. Look for dehiscence of lamina papyracea.
5. Look for abnormal cells such as Onodi and Haller cells.
6. Look for bony erosions: these can be due to:
   a. Previous surgery
   b. Mucocele or mass
   c. Developmental
7. Look for changes due to disease
   a. Acute sinusitis can cause a fluid level. Air fluid level is also caused by blood in the sinus following an antral lavage/cerebraspinal fluid (CSF) leak.
   b. Chronic sinusitis:
      1. Diffuse or polypoidal mucosal thickening
      2. Complete opacification
      3. Bone thickening
      4. Polyposis
   c. Fungal sinusitis: focal hyperdense lesion with surrounding hypodense mucoid material. Reactive bony changes are seen. There may also be areas of osteomyelitis.

What is the role of MRI in sinus disease?

Depending on density of secretions:

Watery secretions hypointense on T_1 and hyperintense on T_2

Conventional secretions hypointense on T_2. So if concentration of secretions has 30% of proteins, it will be hypointense on T_1 and T_2 and hence look like normal aerated sinuses.

What are Messerklinger and Wigand techniques?

Messerklinger is an anterior to posterior technique and starts with uncinectomy, ethmoid bulla exposure, frontal sinus ostium, identification of skull base followed by anterior ethmoidectomy, posterior ethmoidectomy and sphenoidectomy.

Wigand is posterior to anterior approach starts with partial middle turbinectomy, opening of posterior ethmoid cells, sphenoid sinus and proceed to anterior ethmoid cells.

Describe the course of anterior ethmoidal artery

It is a branch of the opthalmic artery and passes between the medial and superior rectus muscles. Enters the ethmoid through the anterior ethmoidal foramen. It crosses the ethmoid either at ethmoid roof or up to 5 mm below ethmoid roof. It enters the olfactory area intracranially through lamina cribrosa and re-enters nasal cavity and divides into superior, lateral, medial, and posterior branches.

How frequently will you remove debris from a postoperative cavity?

After initial postoperative debridement on 3rd to 6th day, frequent cleaning is necessary only for patients with extensive polyposis and allergic fungal rhinosinusitis.

What are the complications of FESS?

Hemorrhage from posterior septal artery below sphenoid sinus and middle turbinate arteries.

Orbital complications: Avoiding this involves identifying lamina papyracea which is superior to the maxillary sinus ostia. To identify breach in the lamina papyracea, the lateral wall of the nose should be viewed with the endoscope while the orbit is being palpated.

If there is bleeding from the anterior and posterior ethmoidal arteries resulting in orbital hematoma or raised intraorbital pressure, an immediate lateral canthotomy and cantholysis should be done.

Blindness can result due to increased intraorbital pressure for 60–70 minutes or direct injury to the optic nerve.

Diplopia indicates extraocular muscle injury. Ophthalmic opinion should be sought, but the prognosis is poor. Nasolacrimal duct injury can be avoided by never dissecting anterior to anterior attachment of middle turbinate. If injury has occurred, endoscopic dacryocystorhinostomy (DCR) may be needed.

Intracranial complications:
Dissection along medial aspect of middle turbinate can result in fracture of skull base leading to CSF rhinorrhea. If apparent during surgery, it should be repaired by fascia/cartilage/fat grafts.

Delayed leaks may be identified by endoscopy, CT cisternogram or intrathecal injection of flourescien and endoscopy. Leaks which are small heal by 2–3 weeks; if not, it has to repaired.

What is Kero's classification?

Depends on the depth of the olfactory fossa.
Type I—1-3 mm
Type II—4-7 mm
Type III—8-17 mm

Deeper the fossa, the vertical lamella of the cribriform plate is longer. The increased length of thin bone is more prone to injury. If forceps is used in this region, even a shallow fossa may cause injury. The olfactory fossa is made up of horizontal lamella of cribriform plate medially, the vertical lamella more laterally (0.2 mm thick) and the bony lamella of the frontal bone more laterally (0.5 mm thick).

What are the results of endoscopic polypectomy?

- Only polyps: Good
- Polyps + asthma: Recurrence is higher
- Polyps + asthma + aspirin allergy: Recurrence is highest.

How do steroids help?

It is anti-inflammatory and it also increases apoptosis of inflammatory cells.

What are the boundaries of the frontal recess and how do you approach it?

The frontal recess is bounded medially by the middle turbinate, laterally by the lamina papyracea and anteriorly by the posterior surface of the agger nasi cell. Frontal recess can be approached by removing the remnants of the uncinate process. Superiorly 30° endoscope is helpful to visualize frontal recess and it can be cleared of polyps and disease. The frontal sinus ostia should not be traumatised.

How do you approach the sphenoid sinus ostia endoscopically?

1. Between septum and middle turbinate posteriorly.
2. Lateral to middle turbinate by opening posterior ethmoid cells and exposing superior meatus and turbinate.

The ostium is 7 cm from the anterior end of the nasal cavity at a 30° angle. Sinus can be cleared after widening ostia (but not circumferentially).

How do you avoid optic nerve injury during this procedure?

If there is extensive pneumatization of the sphenoid including anterior clinoid pneumatization, then optic nerve is vulnerable.

There are 4 types of relationship of optic nerve to posterior sinuses.

Type I: Optic nerve causes no indentation of sphenoid or contact with posterior ethmoid air cells (76%).

Type II: Indentation of sphenoid, but no contact with posterior ethmoid air cell.

Type III: Nerve in the sphenoid sinus is surrounded 50% by air.

Type IV: Courses adjacent to both sphenoid and posterior ethmoid cell.

What is the best time to do a CT scan of nose and peripheral nervous system (PNS)?

Medical treatment to reduce mucosal edema gives a more accurate idea of the extent of disease. It could be 3–6 weeks after an inflammatory process.

Spraying the nose with a nasal decongestant may give a more accurate picture.

What anatomical structures can block the osteomeatal complex?

1. Deviated septum.
2. Concha bullosa (aerated middle turbinate).
3. Inverted middle turbinate (paradoxical).
4. Large bulla ethmoidalis.
5. Everted uncinate process.
6. Haller cell (infraorbital cell).
7. Agger nasi cell (obstructs frontal sinus).

What are Onodi cells?

Onodi cell is a posterior ethmoid cell extending lateral and superior to the sphenoid. The optic nerve may be prominent in the lateral wall and may have a dehiscent or thin bony covering.

Describe the various superior attachment of the uncinate process

1. Medially to middle turbinate.
2. Superiorly it can reach skull base.
3. Attached to orbit. In this case infundibulum ends in a blind alley/terminal recess.

Chapter 8

Inverted Papilloma

A 45-year-old man presents with right sided nasal block—1 year.

Mucoid nasal discharge which is occasionally blood tinged from right nasal cavity for 6 months.

HISTORY OF PRESENT ILLNESS

The nasal block has been progressive not relieved by medication or change in posture. It is continuous. Occasionally, there is mucoid nasal discharge from the right nasal cavity which is slightly tinged with blood.
No epistaxis on nose blowing or cleaning of nose.
No other nasal/orbital/ear/throat symptoms.

Slight change in the voice since 3 months. The change is in the quality and there is no difficulty in producing voice or sustaining it.

Nasal block can cause a lack of normal resonance of voice which is sometimes perceived by the patient.

Palatal paralysis also causes a change in voice but this is accompanied by nasal regurgitation.

Rest of history/general examination as usual

On examination

- External nose: Normal
- Vestibule: Normal
- Anterior rhinoscopy: Reveals a mass filling the right nasal cavity with an irregular surface, no ulceration. It is pale pink in color, not pulsatile. No other structures of the lateral wall are visible. Part of septum is seen anteriorly and it is normal. Small amount of discharge is seen in the floor of right nasal cavity.

Left nasal cavity inferior turbinate seen, middle turbinate is visible, nasal mucosa is normal. No discharge is seen in the left nasal cavity.

On probing the mass is soft, not friable, does not bleed on touch and there is space between the mass and the septum. It seems to be arising from the lateral wall.

- Posterior rhinoscopy: Normal
- Oral cavity and oropharynx normal (*look particularly at gingivolabial sulcus for fullness*)
- Orbit is normal. Vision is normal
  Ears/larynx normal
  No neck nodes.

Diagnosis: Benign mass in the nasal cavity?
- ? inverted papilloma.

There is blood stained nasal discharge; Can it occur in benign nasal masses?

1. Benign tumors cause obstruction to airflow and so crusting results in necrosis causing bleeding.
2. Patient may blow nose harder to relieve obstruction and crusting resulting in bleeding.
3. Self digital cleaning of crusts also results in blood stained discharge.

Can benign masses cause pain?

Yes.
1. Due to sinonasal block/rhinosinusitis.
2. Dural or orbital contact.
3. Pain may be due to some other cause and a CT for diagnosis of pain may reveal an incidental benign mass.

What are the symptoms of benign nasal tumors?

Benign tumors may be symptom-less or initial symptoms may later on be ignored. This is because of adaptation to symptoms, i.e. worsening of impairment of function with decreased symptom awareness.

Benign tumors may grow over a long time and suddenly cause symptoms because of associated viral infection.

There may be persistent postnasal drip.

Pain/bleeding.

Orbital symptoms and loss of olfaction is rare in benign tumors.

How will you classify benign tumors?

For practical purposes, it can be divided into:
1. Fibro-osseous
   - Fibrous dysplasia
   - Chondroma
   - Osteoma.
2. Inverted papilloma.
3. Nerve related
   - Schwannoma

- Neuroma
- Meningioma
- Chordoma.

4. Vascular
   - Juvenile nasopharyngeal angiofibroma.
5. Odontogenic ameloblastoma.

What do you think this is?

Inverted papilloma.
It is also classified as intermediate tumor (between benign and malignant).

Why do you think it is inverted papilloma?

It is the commonest tumor of the sinonasal tract. It can be of 3 types:

a. Septal (fungiform)
b. Inverted
c. Oncocytic (cylindrical).

It forms less than 5% of tumors of nose/PNS, but it is frequently encountered because

1. Potential for growth
2. Recurrence
3. Malignant change.

It is a differential diagnosis for polyps as it is associated with polyps. It occurs as a nodular papillomatous, unilateral mass.

Histopathologically, there is thickened squamous epithelium, mixed chronic inflammatory exudates, downward growth into a fibromyxoid stroma. There is osteitis within the mass to denote the site of origin and also osteitis at the site of bony attachment

Why should bone be resected in inverted papilloma?

Pseudopods extend into the bone and hence bony resection is necessary.

What histopathological changes denote malignancy?

Atypia, dysplasia, carcinoma in situ and squamous cell carcinoma are all seen. 9.1% undergo malignant change. The histopathological change which can most probably denote premalignant change is carcinoma in situ.

How will you treat the patient?

Patient needs a diagnostic endoscopy and biopsy. Prior to this a CT scan will show the extent of tumor and bony destruction.

Following this the mass can be resected endoscopically by doing a medial maxillectomy.

A lateral rhinotomy approach and a medial maxillectomy is the second option.

Limited resection is not advisable.

Recurrence rate:
Endoscopic removal—12.8%
Lateral rhinotomy—17.0%
Limited resection—34.2%.

What is medial maxillectomy?

Through a lateral rhinotomy incision a block of bone consisting of the lateral nasal wall, including all turbinate tissue and contents of maxillary and ethmoid sinuses are removed. The lamina papyracea is also removed.

This cannot be used for tumors extending to orbit, anterior cranial fossa, anterolateral wall of maxilla or alveolus.

Complication is epiphora.

What can be done for alveolar or palatal tumors?

Partial maxillectomy involving removal of lower half of maxilla.

What are the other common benign tumors of nose and PNS?

Hemangioma: Lobular papillary hemangioma is the commonest and is synonymous with pyogenic granulation and vascular pregnancy tumors.

It arises as a reddish purple lobulated swelling on the septum or inferior turbinate in young people.

Osteoma and fibro-osseous dysplasia: Osteoma is present in 1% of all radiographs in 3-4 decade of life. It is common in the frontal and ethmoidal sinuses. It presents as a smooth, mucosal covered mass. Ivory osteoma has hard dense bone with few fibrous components. It is difficult to drill.

Fibrous dysplasia: It can be monostotic or polyostotic. Radiologically, it has a ground glass appearance.

Odotogenic cysts:
Radicular cyst occurs as a result of a periapicular infection.
Dentigerous cyst occurs around an unerupted tooth.
Odontogenic kerato cyst: It is benign but an aggressive cyst arising from the dental lamina which is a band of epithelial tissue seen in histological sections of a developing tooth.
Ameloblastoma is also of odontogenic origin

What are the syndrome associated with benign tumors of the nose and PNS?

1. Gardner's syndrome:
    - Osteoma
    - Colorectal polyposis
    - Supernulmerary teeth
    - Skeletal abnormalities.

2. Gorlin's syndrome:
    - Odontogenic keratocyst
    - Basal cell carcinoma
    - Skeletal abnormalities.
3. McSune Albright syndrome:
    - Polyostotic fibrous dysplasia
    - Cafe-au-lait spots
    - Endocrine abnormalities.

What is the role of CT/MRI in benign sinonasal masses?

1. Soft tissue changes fill sinuses where it is difficult to differentiate between secretions/tumors.
2. Bony changes are usually pressure induced and can cause bony expansion.

    CT opacity indicates:
    1. Tumor
    2. Mucocele
    3. Encephalocele
    4. Intracranial extension

    MRI is indicated:
    1. Skull base erosion
    2. Orbital erosion
    3. Frontal sinus involvement.

Chapter

9

Sinonasal Malignancy

A 50-year-old man presents with blood stained nasal discharge from right nasal cavity 3 months duration;

Protrusion of the right eye—15 days.

HISTORY OF PRESENT ILLNESS

The blood stained nasal discharge started three months ago and was occasional, only once in 2–3 days followed by more frequent blood stained discharge. Now every time patient blows his nose the discharge is blood stained. He also complains of increased nasal discharge which is mucoid from the right nasal cavity.

Nasal block is unilateral present on the right side, present all the time and has been increasing progressively over 3 months. Over the past 15 days, he noticed that his right eye is more prominent than the left eye. There is no loss of vision, double vision, and redness of the eye, itching or pain. The left eye is symptomless. There is no unexplained falling or loosening of the teeth. Patient does not wear dentures.

(Maxillary sinus malignancies involving the alveolar margin cause widening of alveolar margin and may also cause erosion of bone. This results in dentures which do not fit or teeth which loosen)

- No history of headache or facial pain.
  (*Involvement of the trigeminal nerve causes facial anesthesia, paresthesia or facial pain*)
  (*Headache may results from blocked sinus or from intracranial involvement*)
- No history of trismus
  (*Involvement of the muscles of mastication in the infra temporal fossa can cause trismus*)
- No history of ear pain, ear discharge or hard of hearing.
  (*Ear involvement may be secondary to extension into nasopharynx and eustachian tube involvement. Otalgia can be refined otalgia*)
- No history of sneezing
- No history of anosmia/hyposmia.

Patient has undergone treatment for nasal discharge and nasal block where he was prescribed nasal drops and antibiotics.

Past history: No history of tuberculosis, diabetes or hypertension.

Patient has not been associated with the wood industry or any chemical industry or watch making industry.
(Hard wood workers are likely to develop adenocarcinoma whereas people working with soft wood can have squamous cell carcinoma. Wood particles inhibit ciliary movement and cause irritation due to presence of wood particles. Nickel, chromium, paint, radium dial painting on watches can also be etiological factors for sinonasal malignancies. African mahogany is one of the important causes for carcinoma of the nose and sinuses)

Patient is not a smoker or alcoholic (*not significant in this malignancy*).

General examination: To be done as in all cases.
Rate malignancy patients on the Eastern Cooperative Oncology Group scale.

ENT examination
- External nose shows widening in the region of the right nasal bone. No other abnormality seen. No facial swelling
- Vestibule: Blood stained discharge is seen in the right nasal vestibule, left nasal vestibule is normal
- **Anterior rhinoscopy:**
  - *Right nasal cavity:* An ulceroproliferative mass is seen filling the nasal cavity. It is reddish pink in color, turbinates, roof, floor are not seen. Mass when probed is soft, bleeds slightly, and appears attached to the lateral wall, there is space between the septum and the mass for the probe to pass through. Mass is not pulsatile.
  - Left nasal cavity mucosa normal over septum, lateral wall and floor. Inferior turbinate is normal minimal secretions are seen on the floor of the nasal cavity which is mucoid and not blood stained.
- **Posterior rhinoscopy:** Posterior end of the septum is seen. Ulceroproliferative mass is visible through the right choana but not filling it. The upper part of the right choana is free. Left choana, eustachian tube orifice, fossa of Rosen-muller, roof of nasopharynx are normal.
- **Examination of the oral cavity:** Lips, angle of the mouth, vestibule of the mouth is normal, gingvolabial sulcus is free. Alveolar ridges are normal.
- Dentition loss of II molar on the left upper jaw. Poor oral hygiene
- No palatal bulge
- Palatal movements are normal
- **Oropharynx:** Normal
- **IDL scopy:** No abnormality seen. Both cords normal in structure and mobility
- **Ears:** No abnormality seen
- **Examination of the eye:** The right eye ball is pushed outwards and laterally. Movements of the extraocular muscles normal. Patients vision is apparently normal
- Examination of cranial nerves II, III, IV, V and VI are normal.

How does extension to orbit occur?

It can occur through the roof of maxilla, the ethmoid sinus, through the pterygomaxillary fossa, and infraorbital fissure.
Examination of the neck: No palpable neck nodes.
Laryngeal architecture is normal.

Diagnosis: Sinonasal malignancy.
Probably maxillary because 70% of malignancies of the nose and sinuses is in the maxilla.
(20% ethmoid, 3% sphenoid, 1% frontal).

What is the stage?

T_3 No Mx.

Describe TNM/Staging of maxillary malignancies

TNM staging of nasal cavity and paranasal sinuses:
- Primary tumor (T)
- Tx primary tumor cannot be assessed
- To No evidence of tumor
- T_{1s} carcinoma is situ.

Maxillary sinus:
- T_1 tumor limited to maxillary sinus mucosa with no erosion or bony destruction
- T_2 tumor causing bone erosion or destruction including extension into the hard palate and/or middle meatus except extension to posterior wall of maxillary sinus or pterygoid plates
- T_3 tumor invades any of the following, bone of posterior wall of maxilla, subcutaneous tissue, floor of medial wall of orbit, pterygoid fossa, and ethmoid sinuses
- T_{4a} moderately advanced local disease. Tumor invades anterior orbital contents, skin of cheek, pterygoid plates, infratemporal fossa, cribriform plate, sphenoid or frontal sinuses
- T_{4b} very advanced local disease. Tumor invades any of the following: Orbital apex, dura, brain, middle cranial fossa, cranial nerves other than maxillary division of V, nasopharynx or clivus.

T staging of nasal cavity and ethmoid sinus:
- T_1 tumor limited to any one subsite with or without bony invasion
- T_2 tumor invading two subsites in a single region or extending to involve an adjacent region within the nasoethmoidal complex with or without bony invasion
- T_3 Tumor extends to involve the medial wall or floor of orbit, maxillary sinus, palate or cribriform plate
- T_{4a} Moderately advanced local disease. Tumor invades any of the following: Anterior orbital contents, skin of nose or cheek, minimal

extension to anterior cranial fossa, pterygoid plates, sphenoid or frontal sinuses.

- T_{4b} very advanced local disease: Tumor invades any of the following: Orbital apex, dura, brain, middle cranial fossa, cranial nerves other than (V2), nasopharynx, clivus.

Regional lymph nodes: N

- Nx regional lymph nodes cannot be assessed
- N_0 any regional lymph node metastasis
- N_1 metastasis in a single ipsilateral lymph node, 3 cm or less in greatest dimension
- N_2
- N_{2a} Metastasis in a single ipsilateral lymph node more than 3 cm but less than 6 cm in greatest dimension
- N_{2b} metastasis into multiple ipsilateral lymph nodes none more than 6 cm in greatest dimension
- N_{2c} metastasis in bilateral or contralateral lymph nodes none more than 6 cm in greatest dimension
- N_3 metastasis in a lymph node more than 6 cm in greatest dimension.

Distant metastasis:

- M_0 no distant metastasis
- M_1 distant metastasis
- Mx distant metastasis cannot be assessed.

Staging:

- Stage 0: $T_{1s}N_0M_0$
- Stage 1: $T_1 N_0 M_0$
- Stage II: $T_2 N_0 M_0$
- Stage III: $T_1/T_2 N_1 M_0$
- $T_3 N_0$
- $T_3 N_1$
- Stage IV A $T_{4a} N_0 M_0$
- $T_{4a} N_1 M_0$
- $T_1 T_2 T_3 T_{4a} N_2 M_0$
- Stage IV B T_{4b} Any N M_0
- Any T $N_3 M_0$
- Stage IV C Any T, Any N M_1.

What are the subsites of the nasal cavity?

i. Septum
ii. Floor
iii. Lateral wall
iv. Vestibule.

What is the histological grading?

- Gx grade cannot be assessed
- G_1 well differentiated

- G_2 moderately differentiated
- G_3 poorly differentiated
- G_4 undifferentiated.

What is the lymphatic drainage of this region?

Primary spread to retropharyngeal node and later to upper jugular nodes. Soft tissue of face and skin drains to submandibular node and later to upper jugular node. Distant metastasis is rare.

What are the investigations?

1. CT and MRI

   CT detects bony erosion of
   - Bony orbital wall
   - Cribriform plate
   - Fovea ethmoidalis
   - Posterior wall of maxilla
   - Pterygopalatine fossa
   - Sphenoid sinus
   - Posterior table of frontal bone.

   Coronal cuts good for orbital floor and skull base, cribriform plate.
   Axial cuts good for posterior wall of maxilla, pterygopalatine fossa, infratemporal fossa.

   CT cannot say whether periorbita has been breached. It cannot differentiate tumor from soft tissue and secretions. Contrast may help.

   In the orbital apex, there is a central low density area of fat surrounding optic nerve and a radial arrangement of extraocular muscles. Loss of this plane implies advanced disease because veins in this region have direct access to the cavernous sinus.

   CT can also assess nasopharyngeal infiltration. Thickening of the normal thin layer of mucosa covering the medial pterygoid plate denotes infiltration.

   MRI: Differentiates tumor from secretions and soft tissue. Inflammation and secretions give low intensity images with T_1, and high intensity images with T_2 because of increased water content. Sinonasal tumors are 95% cellular and so low on water content, so there is low to intermediate intensity images with T_1 and T_2

   With gadolinium enhancement:

   Tumors enhances in a diffuse manner to an intermediate degree. Inflamed mucosa enhances intensely and in a peripheral manner.

   MRI also delineates perineural spread in adenoid cystic carcinoma.
2. Diagnostic nasal endoscopy followed by biopsy avoid anterior antrostomies for biopsy as there will be seeding of gingivolabial sulcus and skin of cheek with tumor.

3. Dental opinion for oral sepsis and obturator following surgery.
4. Ophthalmic opinion.
5. X-ray chest.

How do tumors spread from maxilla?

- Medial—nose
- Inferior—inferior alveolar margin
- Posterior—infratemporal fossa
  pterygomaxillary fossa.

From pterygomaxillary fossa tumor can spread by the following routes:

a. Foramen rotundum to middle cranial fossa
b. Pterygoid canal to foramen lacerum
c. Sphenopalatine foramen to nasopharynx
d. Pterygomaxillary fissure to infratemporal fossa
e. Infraorbital fissure to orbital apex.

- Lateral—To form a mass below the orbit
- Anterior—To soft tissue of cheek.

What is Ohngren's Line?

It is a line drawn from the medial canthus of the orbit to the angle of the mandible. Malignant tumors above this line may have worse prognosis. This was true before the advent of craniofacial resection.

What is the treatment protocol for maxillary sinus tumor?

- T_{1-2} No
- All histologies except adenoid cystic carcinoma: Complete resection. If the margins are negative—follow up
- If there is perineural invasion: CTRT
- If margins are positive—repeat surgery. Following surgery if margins are negative—RT is enough. If margins are positive—CTRT is needed
- In adenoid cystic carcinoma T_1 T_2 no complete resection followed by:
  - If suprastructure is involved—RT
  - If infrastructure—follow up/RT
- In T_3-T_{4a} No: For squamous cell carcinoma complete resection followed by CTRT to primary/neck if margins are positive
- If there are no adverse features then only RT to primary/neck
- In T_{4b} and any N CTRT is the choice.

In T_1-T_{4a} N^+: Resection + neck dissection. If margins are free RT to primary and neck is enough. If there are adverse features then CTRT to neck and primary is needed.
(Adverse features include positive margins and extracapsular spread in the nodes.)

What is postoperative RT?

- Primary 60–66 Gy (2.0/Gy/fraction)
- Neck
  Involved nodes 60–66 Gy (2.0 Gy/fraction)
  Uninvolved nodes 44–64 Gy (1.6 to 2.0 Gy/fraction)
- IMRT is preferred technique for paranasal tumors.

What is the treatment protocol for ethmoid sinus tumors?

- T_1T_2—surgical excision. This is followed by RT if margins are free or by CTRT if there are adverse features
- T_3 T_{4a} Surgical excision followed by CTRT
- T_{4b} CTRT
- If diagnosed after surgical procedures like polypectomy, if gross residual disease persists—surgical excision—CTRT
- No gross residual disease—RT.

What are types of radiotherapy for maxillary tumors?

- Definitive RT
- For primary and gross adenopathy
  a. Conventional fractionation: 66–74 Gy
     (2.0 Gy/fraction daily for 5 days a week)
  b. Altered fractionation
     66–74 Gy/primary/6 fractions per week
  c. Concomitant boost accelerated RT
     72 Gy/6 weeks (1.8 Gy/fraction large field with 1.5 Gy boost as a second daily fraction during the last 12 days of treatment)
  d. Hyperfractionation 81.6 Gy/7 weeks
     (1.2 Gy/fraction twice daily)

- Uninvolved neck 44–64 Gy (1.6 Gy–2.0 Gy/fraction)
- Postoperative RT
- Primary 60–66 Gy (2.0 Gy/fraction)
- Neck nodes + 60–66 gy (2.0 Gy fraction)
- Nodes negative 44–64 Gy
  (1.6–2.0 Gy/fraction).

What will you do for this patient?

Total maxillectomy with postoperative radiotherapy for primary and neck.

If there are adverse features than CTRT will have to be given postoperatively.

What is total maxillectomy?

Preoperative workup includes:

1. Ophthalmic opinion

2. Prosthodontic consultation for primary obturator
   Incisions: Weber Ferguson's incision for the skin. A buccal incision is made in the upper buccal sulcus up to maxillary tuberosity. A palatal incision is made from the incision to the junction of the hard and soft palate. Both buccal and palatal incisions meet around the tuberosity. Exposure is gained by making a full thickness flap. Further the orbital floor is exposed and periostium separated from bone. The lacrimal sac and inferior orbital fissure are identified. The pterygomaxillary fissure is exposed.

   This is followed by osteotomies which are 6 in numbers:
   1. Frontal process of maxilla.
   2. Nasal bone.
   3. Through the zygomaticomaxillary suture from inferior orbital fissure to pterygomaxillary fissure.
   4. Orbital floor.
   5. Pterygomaxillary fissure.
   6. Palatal suture usually cut with Gigli saw. Rest of the bones can be separated by chisel.

- Specimen is removed by rocking. Bleeding may be noticed now due to involvement of terminal branch of maxillary artery or done to pterygoid plexus of veins.
- Cavity is lined by split skin grafts
- Cavity is packed with Bismuth, Iodine, and Paraffin Paste (BIPP) pack and an obturator left in situ.
- This is total maxillectomy as all the walls are removed.

How will you manage the orbit?

Orbital exenteration is indicated if there is:
1. Involvement of orbital apex.
2. Involvement of extraocular muscles.
3. Involvement of bulbar conjunctive or sclera.
4. Lid involvement.
5. Involvement of retro orbital fat.

What are the contraindications for surgical excision of mass?

1. Distant metastasis.
2. Extensive intracranial involvement.
3. Bilateral cavernous sinus involvement.
4. Disease involving both orbits.

Are there any procedures for more extensive disease?

Craniofacial resection can be done when there is extension to roof of ethmoid or involvement of orbital apex, pterygoid region.

A lateral rhinotomy incision is extended to expose:

1. Frontal sinus.
2. Floor of anterior cranial fossa.
3. Ethmoid labyrinth (exentration of orbit when required).
4. Nasal septum. This procedure gives direct exposure to cribriform plate and fovea ethmoidalis. Dural tears can be repaired.

Extended craniofacial resection is tailor made to remove structure such as pteryogid plates, sphenoid sinus and can extend up to foramen ovale posteriorly. Even if this resection is made there may not be clear margins particularly at the pterygoid space, orbital apex, and nasopharynx.

What are the other malignant tumors of nose and PNS other than squamous cell carcinoma?

Epithelial

i. Adenocarcinoma
ii. Transitional cell carcinoma
iii. Salivary gland tumor
iv. Anesthesio-neuroblastoma.

Non-epithelial

i. Fibrosarcoma
ii. Angiosarcoma
iii. Hemangiosarcoma
iv. Chondrosarcoma
v. Osteogenic sarcoma
vi. Plasmacytoma.

What is Anesthesio-neuroblastoma?

This tumor is seen in the olfactory region of the nose (cribriform plate). It can occur in the second or fifth decade of life. It is commoner in women. It is a neuroendocrine tumor. It can range from an indolent mass to an extremely aggressive tumor.

Kadish has classified it as:

a. Limited to nose
b. Present in nasal cavity and sinuses
c. Extension beyond nasal cavity and sinuses
d. Extension to cervical nodes and distant sites.

Best treatment is surgical excision followed by CTRT.

Chapter 10

Nasopharyngeal Angiofibroma

A 15-year-old boy presents with Nasal block—1 year, Epistaxis—1 year.

Nasal block is present for the past one year, gradually progressive, present all the time, in both nasal cavities.

It is accompanied by nasal discharge which is mucoid and occasionally blood stained. Nasal discharge occurs intermittently. There is no history of sneezing, headache, anosmia, itching along the nasal ala or medial canthus of the eye, no watering of eyes.

Epistaxis occurs spontaneously, is profuse and self limiting. He has had 3-4 episodes per year, has been admitted once and nasal packing was done. Patient complains of protrusion of right eye since two months, vision is normal, no history of double vision.

- No history of unexplained falling of teeth
- No history of swelling over the cheek
- No history of trismus
- No history of loss of sensation over face or facial pain (*due to involvement of V cranial nerve*)
- No history of difficulty in swallowing, aspiration, nasal regurgitation
- (*Due to involvement of last four cranial nerves)*
- Patient has a plummy voice, nasal intonation is lost
- No history of fever
- No history of ear symptoms.

Past history: No history of tuberculosis
Family history: Not significant
Personal history: Vegetarian/not a smoker/nonalcoholic.

From the history what do you think it is?

Because of male sex, bilateral nasal block, spontaneous epistaxis, age and proptosis.

It may be a benign swelling of the nasopharynx.

What benign swelling do you expect?

As it is a young boy presenting with epistaxis it could be a nasopharyngeal angiofibroma.

Can it be malignancy?

Sometimes nasopharyngeal carcinoma has a bimodal presentation but there is no cervical lymphadenopathy or cranial nerve involvement.

Clinical examination

External nose: Bridge of the nose is widened on the right side, no swelling over the face.
Vestibule is normal.
Anterior rhinoscopy reveals mucoid discharge both nasal cavities. There is a whitish opaque mass seen in the posterior part of the right nasal cavity. It cannot be probed. The surface is smooth. It occupies the whole of the posterior part of the right nasal cavity. In the floor of the nasal cavity mucoid secretions which is blood tinged is seen. Left nasal cavity shows secretion in the nasal cavities, mucoid in nature, no other abnormality seen.

Septum is in the mid line.

Posterior rhinoscopy reveals a pinkish white mass in the nasopharynx occupying all of the nasopharynx except a small portion of the choana laterally on the left side.

Eustachian tube orifices are not seen

Surface of the swelling is smooth with few petechia, posterior end of the septum not seen.

Oral cavity: normal except that the soft palate is pushed downwards on the right side. Palatal movements are normal.

Ear both tympanic membrane normal.

Tunning fork tests do not reveal any hearing loss.

Indirect laryngoscopy: Posterior third of tongue, vallecula, epiglottis, ventricular fold, vocal cords normal, pyriform fossa no pooling of saliva or mass seen.

Neck: No palpable mass/no other abnormality seen.

Examination of eyes:

- *Right eye:* Proptosis present, movements of extraocular muscles normal. No apparent loss of vision.
- Left eye is normal.

What is your Diagnosis?

Benign mass in the nasopharynx—nasopharyngeal angiofibroma.

What are other benign swelling in the nasopharynx?

- Adenoids
- Thornwaldt's and mucosal cysts
- Choanal polyps
- Fibroma
- Papilloma

- Osteoma
- Fibrous dysplasia.

Some tumors present in the nasopharynx
- Craniopharyngioma
- Extracranial meningioma
- Chordoma.

All salivary gland tumors except Warthin's can occur. Commonly seen are adenoid cystic carcinoma and pleomorphic adenoma.

What is the site of origin of nasopharyngeal angiofibroma?

Superior margin of the sphenopalatine foramen formed by palatine bone, horizontal ala of vomer and root of pterygoid process.

How does nasopharyngeal angiofibroma extend?

From the sphenopalatine foramen it can axtend anteriorly into the nasal cavity.
It can extend posteriorly into the nasopharynx.

It can spread laterally through pterygomaxillary fissure to infratemporal fossa, curve around posterior wall of maxilla and present as a cheek swelling.

It can extend to maxillary, ethmoid and sphenoid sinuses.

Superior: It extends to middle cranial fossa through roof of the infratemporal fossa or superior orbital fissure. Here, it may be lateral to cavernous sinus and anterolateral to internal carotid artery.

It can spread to superior orbital fissure and give rise to superior orbital fissure syndrome. It can extend to orbit through the inferior orbital fissure. It invades apex of orbit.

Less commonly it can spread through sphenoid sinus to the sella turcica and occupy a position medial to internal carotid artery and lateral to pituitary gland.

Describe the histopathology of angiofibroma

It has 2 cellular components.
1. Spindle or stellate shaped cells in a dense collagen matrix.
2. Vessels which can be small endothelial lined capillaries to large venous channels.

No smooth muscle or elastic tissue coat.

Depending on components if it is predominantly angiomatous the swelling is soft and bleeds easily, it is fibromatous it can be firm and rubbery.

What are the investigations?

- CT/MRI with contrast
- Anterior bowing of posterior maxillary wall,

- Erosion of bony structures such as sphenoid, hard palate, medial wall of maxillary sinus
- Avoid transantral biopsy as it can cause severe bleeding
- Angiography helps to determine blood supply to tumor and embolization prior to surgery.

How will you stage angiofibroma?

It is staged by

a. Fisch
b. Chandler
c. Session
d. Radkowski.

a. Fisch is the best as it shows how the tumor can be resected.

Fisch

1. Limited to nasopharynx with bone destruction limited to sphenopalatine foramen
2. Tumor invading pterygomaxillary fissure or maxilla, ethmoid or sphenoid with bone destruction
3. Tumor invading infratemporal fossa
   a. Without intracranial extension
   b. With intracranial extension which is extradural
4. Intracranial intradural
   a. Without cavernous sinus/pituitary fossa/or optic chiasma
   b. With involvement of cavernous sinus/pituitary fossa/or optic chiasma.

b. Chandler's staging:

1. Limited to nasopharynx
2. Extending to nose and sphenoid sinus
3. Spread to antrum, ethmoid sinus, pterygomaxillary fossa/infratemporal fossa/orbit/cheek
4. Intracranial extension.

c. Session's classification

IA—Nose and nasopharynx
IB—Extension to one or more sinuses
IIA—Minimal invasion of pterygomaxillary fissure
IIB—Full occupation of pterygomaxillary fissure +– orbit
IIC—Infratemporal fossa/+ cheek extension
III—Intracranial.

d. Radkowski's classification

IA—IB IIA IIB are/classification same as session's
IIC—Infratemporal fossa without cheek extension or pterygoid plates involvement
IIIA—Erosion of skull base/minimal erosion of intracranial fossa
IIIB—Erosion of skull base/extension intracranially + cavernous sinus.

What is the role of preoperative embolization?

- For small tumors, it is not needed
- For extensive tumors embolization followed by surgery within 48 hours
- Embolization reduces blood loss but increases recurrence rate may be because shrinkage of tumor following embolization reduces adequate removal.
- Embolization is necessary prior to endoscopic removal and also for tumors with intracranial extension.

What are the various approaches to nasopharyngeal angiofibroma?

1. Endoscopic removal is indicated for Fisch I, II and some III (where there is limited medial invasion of infratemporal fossa. An anterior ethmoidectomy followed by removal of medial wall of maxillary sinus, gives access to posterior wall of maxillary sinus. Posterior wall is removed to see lateral extent of tumor. Dissect into sphenoid till rostrum is reached. Bipolar cautery and ligaclips for feeding vessels is a must.
2. More extensive tumors need a midfacial degloving. Here anterolateral, medial wall and posterior wall of maxilla can be removed, extension to inferior part of orbit and infratemporal fossa can also be removed.
3. Intracranial extension needs a combined skull base approach. Subtemporal preauricular infratemporal fossa approach with a middle cranial fossa craniotomy.
4. Transpalatine approach was used prior to the advent of endoscopy, it gives access to anterior nasopharynx but limited access to lateral nasopharynx from which angiofibroma arises.
5. Transmaxillary; Here incision is made from tuberosity to tuberosity and osteotomy to fracture alveolus downwards.

How will you treat recurrence?

- Regardless of approach 25% of tumors recur. Younger patients have increased recurrence. Removal of basisphenoid reduces recurrence.
- Depending on the extent of recurrence surgery is repeated. It is the best option.
- It will result in atropic changes of nasal mucosa, injury to nerves, etc.
- Radiotherapy only if surgery cannot be done.
- IMRT may help resolve some problems of external beam irradiation. Irradiation effect takes almost 2 years to resolve.

Chapter 11

Nasopharyngeal Carcinoma

A 50-year-old man presents with history of swelling right side of neck—3 months.

Blood stained nasal discharge right nasal cavity—2 months.

HISTORY OF PRESENT ILLNESS

Swelling in the right side of the neck near the angle of mandible (jaw) started 3 months ago and gradually increased to the size of a lemon. It is painless. The patient noticed blood stained nasal discharge which was occasional 2 months ago, but is more frequent now. The last bout occurred yesterday.

- No history of nasal block
- No history of abnormality of smell
- No history of sneezing, watering of the eyes, itching along ala nasi or medial canthus of eye
- No history of facial pain or paresthesia over the face
- No history of headache
  (Referred pain may be present due to involvement of terminal branches of V Cranial nerve in the nasopharyx). V Cranial nerve involvement due to erosion of skull also causes pain.
- No history of fever
- No ear symptoms such as otalgia or tinnitus or hard of hearing
- No history of visual problems;
- Proptosis or ophthalmoplegia *(due to involvement of orbit)*
  Diplopia *(due to VI Cranial nerve involvement).*
- No history of hoarseness of voice
  (involvement of IX Cranial nerve)
- No regurgitation of food into the nose *(due to palatal paralysis)*
- No trismus *(due to involvement of muscles of mastication in the infratemporal fossa)*
- No symptoms of Horner's syndrome such as enophthalmos, slight drooping of upper eyelid (pseudoptosis) contraction of pupil (miosis) and absence of sweating on affected side of face (anhydrosis).
  Horner's syndrome is present with last 4 cranial nerve involvement.

(Take negative history as in chapter 10. Take past history, family history and personal history)

- No history of fever, loss of appetite, loss of weight, cough *(to rule out tuberculosis)*
- No other family member has the same problem *(nasopharyngeal carcinoma has a genetic predisposition).*

What is your probable diagnosis?

May be it is a sinonasal or nasopharyngeal malignancy.

Which is more likely?

Due to cervical node involvement, it is more likely to be nasopharyngeal malignancy.

On Examination

External nose and vestibule normal.

Anterior rhinoscopy secretions seen in both nasal cavities purulent and blood stained.

Septum is in the midline. Turbinates are normal. Nasal mucosa is normal. No other abnormality seen.

Posterior rhinoscopy a hyperemic lobulated mass with well defined borders is seen in the right fossa of Rosenmüller measuring 2.5 x 2.5 cm in diameter. The surface of the mass is irregular. It does not move with respiration. Posterior end of septum seen, choana normal, roof of nasopharynx and left fossa of Rosenmüller normal.

Eustachian tube orifice not visualized on the right side, but seen on the left side.

Examination of oral cavity—No palatal paralysis. No paralysis of tongue.

Oropharynx—no pharyngeal paralysis seen.

Indirect laryngoscopy—No vocal cord paralysis.
Examination of the neck—A mass 4 cm in maximum dimension seen in the right jugulodigastric region extending from the anterior border of the sternomastoid muscle along lower border of the mandible. It does not extend to the submandibular region. The angle of mandible and lower border of mandible are palpable.

Anterior border of sternomastoid not clearly palpable in the upper 1/3 on the right side. Tip of lobule of ear not lifted. Post and preauricular region are normal. Lower down swelling extends up to the level of hyoid bone. No other palpable mass in the neck.
Laryngeal architecture is normal.
Boccas sign is present.

Eye—Movements of extraocular muscles normal
(VI N involvement leads to lateral rectus palsy)
(III and IV nerve involvement leads to other extraocular muscle palsy)
(Eye involvement is due to involvement of lateral nasal wall, anterior ethmoid cells, lamina papyracea to orbit).

Examination of cranial nerves: Normal
(VN causes facial pain and parasthesia over face. Involvement of last four cranial nerve's due to erosion of jugular foramen and hypoglossal canal)
Collet Sicard syndrome IX, X, XI, XII
Jugular foramen syndrome IX, X, XI.

Examination of the Ears: Both tympanic membrane normal. Tuning fork test normal.
(A nasopharyngeal mass can mechanically block eustachian tube orifice or it can involve muscles around eustachian tube giving rise to otitis media with effusion.)
(Unilateral otitis media with effusion in an adult should raise suspicion of a nasopharyngeal mass).

Clinical Diagnosis

Nasopharyngeal carcinoma.

Can it present as a lobulated mass?

Yes nasopharyngeal carcinoma can present in 2 ways.
1. Lobulated mass with well defined edges which spreads by lymphatics.
2. Infiltrative mass likely to spread to skull base.

Differential diagnosis:
- Amelanotic melanoma
- Undifferentiated sinonasal mass?

How will you confirm your diagnosis?

Prior to examination of nasopharynx by nasophagoscopy CT MRI is to be done to avoid artifacts in CT MRI. Artifacts occur in the CT MRI if done after biopsy.

1. CT: Good to look for skull base erosion
   It is better than MRI for lymph node enlargement
   MRI with gadolinium and fat suppression gives excellent delineation of soft tissue and tissue planes. Tissue specificity is also good. Coronal plane is taken to show skull base foramina . Axial plane shows retropharyngeal space, pterygomaxillary fossa and infratemporal fossa. In a nasopharyngeal mass, there is lateral displacement of parapharyngeal fat.
   Ultrasound of the neck for neck node enlargement not needed if CT is done.
   PET scan distinguishes between post-irradiation edema and recurrence
2. Serology
   IgA anti-VCA (viral capsid antigen) titer is high. It is not very specific for nasoharyngeal carcinoma—95% sensitivit,y 80–90% specificity

IgA anti EA (early antigen) titer is more specific 95%, specificity 80% sensitivity

In endemic areas;

EBVNA (Epstein Barr virus nuclear antigen) test is done on FNAC/biopsy material using specific monoclonal antibodies. Presence indicates likelihood of nasopharyngeal carcinoma.

Negative result excludes nasopharyngeal carcinoma.

All nasopharyngeal carcinoma cells express Epstein Barr virus encoded latent proteins. So in the process, there is increased RNA intracellularly. If cancer cell stains positive for EBVRNA nasopharyngeal carcinoma is confirmed. Cell free small amounts of EBVDNA can be detected by polymerase chain reaction to look for recurrent nasopharyngeal carcinoma.

3. X-ray chest to look for secondaries, second primary:
   - Imaging of liver for secondaries.
   - Imaging of thoracolumbar vertebra, pelvis, femoral head for secondaries
4. FNAC of the neck node.
5. Examination of nasopharynx/Biopsy
   i. 70–90 degrees transoral retrograde nasopharyngoscope shows fossa of Rosenmüller but choana is not seen.
   ii. Antigrade nasopharyngoscopy can be done using 3.5–3.7 mm flexible fibroscope
   iii. Rigid 0–30 degrees, 4 mm Hopkin's rod can also be used. Deviated nasal septum and polyps makes introduction difficult. To open fossa of Rosenmüller patient says áah,' 'na' and then swallows. This exposes even a small lesion in the fossa of Rosenmüller, left fossa of Rosenmüller is best viewed with the scope in the right nasal cavity and vice versa. Biopsy can be taken after extent of tumor is defined. PET/CT may be useful before taking a biopsy if lesion is not well seen.

Biopsy may reveal:

- Type I keratinizing squamous carcinoma which can be well, moderately or poorly differentiated
- Type II non-keratinizing carcinoma
- Type III undifferentiated carcinoma
- Tumor cell stain positive for cytokeratin, so it is epithehal in origin.
- WHO has classified type II and III as subtypes of II
- Type II is common in endemic areas and is Epstein Barr virus related
- Type I is less aggressive, but it is also less radiosensitive. So prognosis worse for type I.

Why do you feel there is a genetic predisposition for nasopharyngeal carcinoma?

1. High incidence among Southern Chinese.
2. High incidence among Southern Chinese immigrants settled in low incidence areas.
3. Low incidence in population with low risk living in high incidence areas, for example: Indians in Singapore.

4. Familial clustering among relatives.
5. Factors like salted fish affects some population like Southern Chinese but Japanese are spared.

Describe the genetic factors

HLA (human leucocytic antigen) is associated with nasopharyngeal carcinoma. The loci involved are HLA, A—B-DR on the short arm of chromosome 6.

Alleles for HLA antigen vary with different population.

- A_2 A_{33} B_{46} B_{58} Cw_1, DR_3 are associated with nasopharyngeal carcinoma
- A_2 Cw_1, B_{46} have highest risk (3.5)
- A_2 Cw_1, B_{46} indicates onset of nasopharyngeal carcinoma above 30 years of age.
- A_{33} Cw_3 B_{58} DR_3 this combination indicates younger age of onset and so poor survival. The relative risk for nasopharyngeal carcinoma
- 1.5 for A_2
- 1.9 for B_{46}
- 2.1 for B_{58}.

People with some of these haplotypes may not be able to develop immunity for nasopharyngeal carcinoma whereas in non-susceptible people when HLA molecules presents antigen to T cells, there is a response to Epstein Barr virus.

Genetically susceptible people have deletion of short area of chromosome 3 and 9. This may be the location of tumor suppressor gene for nasopharyngeal carcinoma.

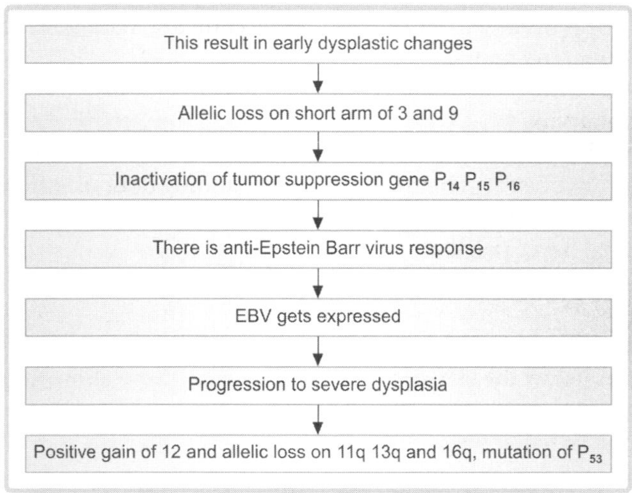

(EBV infection occurs early in life during weaning. Virus is latent in epithelial cells and B lymphocytes)

Describe environmental factors responsible for nasopharyngeal carcinoma

The current thinking is that ingestants may be more responsible than inhalants.

Diet high in salted fish, low in vitamins from fruits and vegetables are more prone.

Volatile nitroamines which are alkylating agents induce malignant charges. Consumption of shrimp paste, salted vegetables also increases risk. Emigrant Chinese continue to consume salted fish.

Describe fossa of rosenmüller

It lies in the lateral wall of the nasopharynx. The eustachian tube opening is triangular in shape. The anterior wall joins the soft palate and the posterior wall is prominent and mobile. To provide place for the posterior wall there is a lateral extension of the nasopharynx lying above and behind the eustachian tube orifice. This is the fossa of Rosenmüller. It is a 1.5 mm deep cleft.
The apex of the fossa of Rosenmüller is related to the anterior margin of the carotid canal. V cranial nerve is anterolateral to the apex.
Base of the fossa is an inferior relation of foramen lacerum.
Inferior wall mucosa covers eustachian tube and levator palate muscle.
Posterior wall merges with mucosa over pharyngobasilar fascia.

What stage is the disease in?

T_1N_{1Mx}
Stage II a.

How do you stage nasopharyngeal carcinoma?

Modified Ho's is the best as far as determining choice of treatment is concerned.

- T_1 nasopharynx only
- T_{2n} nasal cavity
- T_{2o} oropharynx
- T_{2P} parapharyngeal space
- T_{3a} bony involvement below skull base including floor of spheroid
- T_{3b} bony involvement of skull base
- T_{3c} cranial nerve palsies
- T_{3p} parapharyngeal region
- N_o nodes
- N_1 nodes above the skin crease at laryngeal cartilage
- N_2 nodes below the skin crease at laryngeal cartilage above supraclavicular region
- N_3 supraclavicular fossa nodes.

Stages

- Stage I :T_1 T_{2n} T_{20} N_0 M_0
- Stage II a : T_1 T_{2n} T_{20} N_1 N_2 M_0
- Stage II b : T_{2p} T_3 T_{3p} N_0 M_0

- Stage III a : T_{2p} T_3 T_{3p} N_1 N_2 M_0
- Stage III b : T_1 T_{2n} T_{2o} N_3 M_0
- Stage IV a : T_{2p} T_3 T_{3p} N_3 M_0
- Stage IV b :M1 (any T any N)

Is there any other method of staging?

- T_1 tumor confined to nasopharynx or tumor extending to nose and oral cavity with no parapharyngeal extension
- T_2 tumor with parapharyngeal extension
- T_3 tumor involves bony structures of skull base + paranasal sinuses
- T_4 tumor with intracranial extension $\pm$ cranial nerve involvement/ hypopharynx/orbit/extension to infratemporal fossa/masticator space
- N_0 no nodes
- N_1 unilateral node/nodes 6 cm or less in greatest dimension above supraclavicular region and or unilateral/bilateral retropharyngeal nodes 6 cm or less in greatest dimension.
- N_2 bilateral nodes 6 cm of less in greatest dimension above supraclavicular region
- N_3 node more than 6 cm in greatest dimension and or supraclavicular region +
- N_3 a more than 6 cm in greatest dimensions
- N_3 b supraclavicular region node.

What is supraclavicular region?

It is described by Ho. It is space bounded by the superior margin of the sternal end of the clavicle, the superior margin of the lateral end of the clavicle and the region where the neck meets the shoulder. This includes caudal portion IV and VB neck node areas.

The staging in the method is as follows:

- Stage I $T_1N_0M_0$
- Stage II $T_1N_1M_0$
  $T_2N_0M_0$
  $T_2N_1M_0$
- Stage III T_1 $T_2N_2M_0$
  $T_3N_0M_0$
  $T_3N_1N_2M_0$
- Stage IVA $T_4N_0M_0$
  $T_4N_1M_0$
  $T_4N_2M_0$
- Stage IVB Any T N_3 M_0
- Stage IVC Any T any N M_1

Even according to this patient has T_1N_1 and it is stage II.

How will you treat the patient?

- $T_1N_0M_0$: Radiotherapy to nasopharynx $\pm$ elective radiotherapy to neck
- $T_1N_{1\text{-}3}$: Cisplatin 100 mg/m^2 on days 1, 22, 43, + radiotherapy 70 Gy to primary and 50 Gy to gross nodal disease and bilateral neck

- If following this, there is residual neck disease—neck dissection
- No residual neck disease—observe.

How will you treat if disease is M_1?

- Any TNM_1 start on platinum base chemotherapy agents.
- Platinum based chemotherapy drugs are gemicitabine, paclitaxel, cisplatin or cerboplatin
- If response is complete follow it with CT RT
- Intensity-Modulated Radiation Therapy (IMRT) is the preferred mode of radiotherapy
- Primary and gross adenopathy 66–70 Gy (2.0 Gy fraction)
- Neck uninvolved nodes—44–64 Gy (1.6 to 2 Gy fraction)
- If recurrent or metastatic carcinoma where platinum therapy has failed
- Cetuximab + carboplatin can be given
- Gemicitabine monotherapy or in combination with cisplatin may also be tried.

How will you treat local recurrence?

1. Repeat radiotherapy/IMRT.
2. Brachytherapy.
3. Stereotaxic radiotherapy.
4. Salvage surgery.

Problems in salvage surgery are

a. Irradiation blurs margins
b. Frozen section is difficult because of bony margins
c. Proximity to skull base and carotid makes wide enbloc resection difficult.

What are the approaches to the nasopharynx?

1. Lateral rhinotomy with medial maxillectomy exposes nasopharynx
2. Midfacial degloving
3. Leforte/osteotomy
4. Maxillary swing
5. Transpalatine approach
6. Mandibular swing.

What is the prognosis for nasopharyngeal carcinoma?

5 years survival rates are:

- Stage I 80–90%
- Stage II 70–80%
- Stage III 40–60%
- Stage IV A and B 20–40%
- Stage IV C 6 months

Close monitoring is essential as most cases recur in the first three years.

What are the complications of irradiation?

1. Xerostomia (can be life long):
   Drugs like amifostin reduces xerostomia when administered along with irradiation. IMRT also reduces radiation to parotid.
2. Oropharyngeal mucositis.
3. Dermatitis.
4. Alopecia of irradiated area: Subacute complications.
5. Otitis media with effusion/acute otitis media/otitis externa (radionecrosis).
6. Olfactory dysfunction.
7. Nasal crusting/adhesions/rhinosinusitis: Late complications.
8. Trismus.
9. Neck stiffness.
10. Osteoradionecrosis of anterior and lateral skull base.
11. Hypothalamic/pituitary dysfunction.
12. Temporal lobe necrosis can occur 10 years after irradiation.
13. Delayed cranial nerve paralysis resulting in dysarthria/dysphagia.
14. Radiation induced malignancies of nose/PNS/oral cavity/oropharynx.

Chapter 12

Oral Cavity

A 35-year-old woman presents with an ulcer in the mouth—3 months duration.

HISTORY OF PRESENT ILLNESS

Ulcer started as a small swelling on the left side of the mouth which later became an ulcer and has been growing larger to attain the present size. It is painless and bleeds a little on touch or when spicy food is eaten. It has been difficult to eat over the past few days because of the increased size of the ulcer.

She was being treated by a local doctor with tablets but now he asked her to see a specialist.

Is there any unexplained dental problem (falling of teeth) non-fitting denture or sharp tooth?

No.

Do you have an ear pain?

No.
Refered otalgia.

Is there trismus ?

No.
This happens due to involvement of medial pterygoid muscle in malignancies. For causes of trismus refer to chapter 13.

Do you have a bad smell in the mouth?

No.
Halitosis (tumor necrosis).

Is there any weight loss?

No.

Is there odynophagia/dysphagia?

Now, because of the size, I am not able to eat properly.

Is there difficulty in speech?

Yes my speech is not very clear now, it is like I have a marble in my mouth.

Is there anesthesia/hypoanesthesia over face?

No.
All these can be symptoms of oral cancer, including patient's complaint of a painless ulcer which bleeds occasionally.

PAST HISTORY

- There is no history of tuberculosis, syphilis or diabetes. Patient has not been treated for anemia.
- Mechanical effects such as a sharp tooth or ill fitting dentures can also cause chronic irritation leading to squamous cell carcinoma.
- Plummer-Vinson's syndrome is a premalignant condition.
- Leukoplakia's seen in tertiary syphilis is an etiological factor.
- Long-term immune suppressors/renal transplant patients, HIV infections can lead to squamous cell carcinoma.
- HIV usually causes oral leukoplakia/Kaposi's tumor.
- **Family history**: Not significant.

PERSONAL HISTORY

Patient chews tobacco and has been doing so for the past 10 to 12 years.

Risk factors in oral cavity malignancies:
Tobacco and alcohol have a synergistic relationship. Smoking causes genetic alteration such as loss of heterozygosity at 3p and q 11q 1B, mutations of P53 expression, chromosomal polysomy.

Non-smoker	*Smoker*
Oral tongue	Larynx
Buccal mucosa	Hypopharynx
Alveolar ridge	Floor of mouth

Reverse smoking causes palatal squamous cell carcinoma.
Areca nut chewing results in buccal mucosa malignancies.
Human papilloma virus has a role to play.
Ultraviolet radiation is a causative factor in lower lip malignancies.
Pipe smoking also causes lip cancer.

GENERAL EXAMINATION

As in all cases.

Examination of Oral Cavity

- Lips and angle of mouth normal.

- Dental hygiene poor.

2212|2122
2212|2122

There is a ulceroproliferative mass in the buccal mucosa on the left side which is about 5 cm in greatest dimension extending in the mucosal surface opposite both upper and lower alveolar margins. It extends up to the gingivolabial sulcus at its lower end but is well within the mucosa at the upper end. Non-ulcerated area is visible beyond the ulcer posteriorly. Surface is irregular and areas of hemorrhage are seen. Movement of tongue is normal.

Tongue, floor of mouth, retromolar trigone, palate, opposite buccal mucosa, appear normal.

Palpation of mass reveals that it is hard in consistency and the skin on the outer aspect is pinchable.

Tongue palpation shows no induration.

Alveolar margins appear free on palpation.

Examination of oropharynx: Tonsillar pillars, tonsil, posterior pharyngeal wall appear normal. No extension of mass into oropharynx seen.

Examination of nose and PNS: No extension of mass seen in the floor of nasal cavity. Maxilla appears normal.

Examination of the neck:
Laryngeal architecture normal. Trachea is in the midline. No palpable mass. No sinuses.

How does oral cancer present?

It can present as an ulceroproliferative mass in any of the subsites of the oral cavity.

1. Floor of mouth.
2. Alveolar margin both maxillary and mandibular.
3. Retromolar trigone.
4. Buccal mucosa.
5. Oral tongue.
6. Palate.
7. Lip.

In the tongue, it can present as a submucosal induration.

It can extend into oropharynx/maxilla.

An edentulous adult is at increased risk of spread to inferior alveolar foramen due to resorption of the mandible.

Lower lip is more likely to be involved than upper lip. It can present as an ulcer with encrustation or an ulceroproliferative mass. Drainage is to the submandibular nodes. Nodal metastasis is late. Bimanual palpation is essential to make out the degree of infiltration.

In oral cancers look for extension into alveolus, maxilla, and the floor of nose. Mental nerve involvement can cause hypoanesthesia. Likelihood of a second synchronous primary has to be ruled out. Synchronous primary is that which occurs within 6 months of first primary, and if seen after 6 months, it is a metachronous primary.

Common site for metachronous primary in an oral cavity or oropharyngeal malignancies is esophagus.

Diagnosis

Malignant lesion of left buccal mucosa with no secondaries clinically.

What is the Stage?

$T_3 N_0 Mx$

Name some benign ulcers of the oral cavity

1. Aphthous ulcer.
2. Tuberculous.
3. Syphilitic.
4. Viral infection such as Herpes zoster/Epstein-Barr virus.
5. Fungal infection.
6. Dermatological diseases such as pemphigus vulgaris.
7. Immune deficiency states.
8. Drug induced.

How do you stage oral cavity malignancies?

Staging in lip/oral cavity carcinoma
Tx: Primary tumor cannot be assessed
T_0: No evidence of tumor
T_{is}: Carcinoma in situ
T_1: Tumor 2 cm or less in greatest dimension
T_2: Tumor greater than 2 cm but not more than 4 cm in greatest dimension
T_3: Tumor more than 4 cm in greatest dimension
T_{4a}: Moderately advanced local disease: Lip tumor invades through cortical bone, inferior alveolar nerve, floor of mouth, skin of face (chin or nose).

Oral cavity tumor invades adjacent structures example through cortical bone to maxilla or mandible, extrinsic muscles of tongue (genioglossus, hyoglossus, styloglossus, palatoglossus) maxillary antrum, skin of face.

T_{4b}: Very advanced local disease
Tumor involves masseteric space, pterygoid plates, skull base, encases internal carotid artery.

TNM Staging

Stage I: $T_1 N_0 M_0$
Stage II: $T_2 N_0 M_0$

Stage III: $T_3 N_0 M_0$
$T_1 N_1 M_0$
$T_2 N_1 M_0$
$T_3 N_1 M_0$
Stage IV A: $T_4N_0N_1N_2M_0$
$T_1T_2T_3N_2$
Stage IV B: Any T N_3 M_0
T_{4b} any N M_0
Stage IV C: Any T
Any N M_1

What are the essential investigations?

Investigations for oral cavity malignancies are:

1. Orthopantogram.
2. CT scan for evaluating extent particularly mandible.
3. MRI for soft tissue extension.
4. X-ray chest: Look for the following:
   Synchronous primary
   Mediastinal nodes/lung metastasis
   Concomitant tuberculosis
   Chronic obstructive lung disease.
5. Examination under anesthesia to see extent of growth and to take a biopsy. Because of the risk of field cancerization, triple endoscopy is needed.
6. Ultrasound neck in select clinically N_0 neck. B wave ultrasonography to assess depth of lesion of tongue.
7. Positron emission tomography to look for recurrent or residual disease, particularly in the post-irradiation cases.
8. Preoperative and pre-radiotherapy workup.
9. Dental prophylaxis particularly prior to radiotherapy.
10. Speech therapy.
11. Nutritional counseling.

How will you treat this patient?

Excision of the primary through a peroral approach and primary closure/ reconstruction with radial forearm free flap. As this is a N_0 neck but T_3, elective neck dissection has to be done on the left side.

Why do you want to do a neck dissection?

The probability of occult cervical lymph node metastasis is likely to be more than 20%. Therefore, it is better to do a neck dissection. But since levels I, II and III have a high risk of metastasis from oral cancer, even a supraomohyoid neck dissection may be sufficient in an N_0 neck.

What are the premalignant conditions for oral cavity malignancies?

Leukoplakia is a white patch in the oral mucosa. It shows abnormal keratinization as opposed to lichen planus. It appears white because keratin is white when wet. Leukoplakia shows hyperkeratosis, parakeratosis and acanthosis.

Hyperkeratosis: Hyperplasia of stratum corneum.

Parakeratosis: Keratinization with presence of nuclei in stratum corneum.

Acanthosis: Epidermal hyperplasia of stratum spinosum.
If leukoplakia shows areas of dysplasia it is more likely to advance to squamous cell carcinoma. Dysplasia indicates increased nuclear to cytoplasmic ratio, loss of polarity, increased mitosis and loss of intracellular adherence. Dysplasia can be moderate or severe.

Leukoplakia is seen along the occlusal line in the buccal mucosa. It can also occur on alveolar mucosa, tongue, lip, palate and floor of mouth.

Erythroplakia is a red mucosal lesion more likely to become malignant as compared to leukoplakia.

Submucosal firbrosis is caused by betel nut chewing and is characterized by increased sensitivity to casien and results in fibrosis. It has a propensity for squamous cell carcinoma.

Lichen planus may be mistaken for leukoplakia. It has a lacy pattern of white striae. It can be premalignant if there is dyskeratosis.

Fordyce's spots and white spongy nevus both resemble leukoplakia but are not premalignant.

Describe buccal carcinoma

- Betel nut chewing and submucous fibrosis are important causative factors.
- Tumor thickness of less than 6 mm has better survival rates.
- Peroral excision is possible. Healing can occur by secondary intention or by using a split skin graft or for large defects a radial forearm myocutaneous flap.

What is the general treatment plan for oral cavity carcinoma?

$T_{1\text{-}2}\,N_0$:

Option 1: Primary excision ± neck dissection→If there are positive nodes with no extracapsular spread-RT is optional
If there is extracapsular spread in the nodes then chemo-RT or re-excision

Option 2: RT/brachy therapy can be given and if there is residual disease then salvage surgery has to be done.

$T_3\,N_o$:
Excision of the primary + neck dissection. If there is residual disease then chemo-RT/salvage surgery can be tried.

T_{4a} Any N:
Excision of primary + neck dissection. If there is residual disease then CTRT.

$T_{1-3}N_{1-3}$:
Excision of primary + neck dissection. If there is residual disease then salvage surgery/CTRT
N_{2C} requires excision of primary with bilateral neck dissection.

Radiotherapy

- Accelerated fraction 1.6 Gy x 3 times daily x 5 weeks 72 Gy
- Hyperfractionation 1.2 Gy x twice daily x 7 weeks
- Accelerated and hyperfractionation may have better locoregional control and hence better survival rates
- Accelerated fraction has high toxicity symptoms.

How will you treat stage IVB and IVc?

- For stages IV_B and IV_c only palliation is possible.
- In advanced disease, if there is poor general conditions and low performance status, only counseling is possible.
- In advanced disease with good general conditions and moderate to good performance status, RT/CT can be given.

What is performance status?

Performance status is assessed by Eastern cooperative oncology groups or Karnofsky status.

0. Fully active can carry out all predisease activities K-90–100
1. Strenous activity restricted/light activity possible K-70–80
2. Can care for self and is ambulatory. No other activity possible K-50–60
3. Only limited self care/confined to chair 50% of the time K-30–40
4. No self care and confined to bed K-10–20

What are the common tumors of the oral cavity?

- Squamous cell carcinoma—90%
- Adenoid cystic carcinoma—5%
- Melanoma/sarcoma/lymphoma—1–2%.

At what stage do patients with oral cancer present?

- 1/3 present as stage I
- 1/3 as stage II
- Of the remaining 1/3
- 2/3 present as stage III
- 1/3 as stage IV.

When is surgery better than radiotherapy?

1. Younger patient.
2. Possibility of second primary.

3. Post-submucous fibrosis.
4. Lesions close to bone.
5. When cosmetically and functionally good result can be expected.

When is radiotherapy better?

1. If surgery causes impairment in function
2. Surgery is technically difficult as in nasopharynx
3. Patient refuses surgery/high-risk patient.

Describe carcinoma tongue

Carcinoma of the tongue. It is usually seen on the lateral surface, rare on the dorsal surface.
Swelling of dorsal surface of the tongue can be amyloidosis, median rhomboid glossitis erosive lichen planus.
A submucosal oral tongue swelling can be squamous cell carcinoma or it can also be leiomyoma, leiomyosarcoma, rhabdomyosarcoma and neurofibroma.

The usual presentation is an ulceroproliferative mass and sometimes it can be submucosal indurated mass. It extends into the musculature of the tongue and hence limits movement of the tongue. It can extend to floor of mouth. There is a high risk of metastasis. Subclinical nodal metastasis is seen in T_1 and T_2.

Bimanual palpation is needed to assess tumor thickness. Thicker tumors are more likely to have nodal metastasis. Surgery is the treatment of choice, brachytherapy can be tried, but there is a high risk of osteoradionecrosis of mandible.

Surgery

- Less than 3 mm partial glossectomy
- 4–9 mm partial glossectomy + 1 to IV selective neck dissection
- >10 mm partial glossectomy + radical neck dissection + postoperative radiotherapy to primary and neck
- Margins of resection should be 1.5 cm for tumors less than 4 cm and less than 1 cm thick. Larger tumors and thicker tumors should have a 2 cm margin.
- Transoral resection is usually possible. If more than 30% of the tongue is resected a radial forearm fasciocutaneous flap is needed for reconstruction. If volume of tongue has to be replaced then anterolateral thigh flap is used. There is controversy as to whether a bulky immobile muscle flap like pectoralis major myocutaneous flap should be used for reconstruction.

Describe carcinoma floor of mouth

Floor of mouth: Pooling of carcinogenic substances in the lingual gutter is seen to be an important factor. Extension to tongue and mandible is possible. Peroral excision and primary closure can be done. If floor of mouth muscles are excised then reconstruction with a radial forearm flap is necessary. In older people a flap can be raised from the angle of mandible to the nasolabial fold. This full thickness graft is used to repair floor of mouth by rotating it inwards. The pedicle can be cut after 3 weeks.

Prognosis in tongue and floor of mouth:

Tumor thickness 0–3 mm 86%—5 year survival rate
4–7 mm 58%
7 mm 52%.

Describe carcinoma involving mandible

This can present as an exophytic growth or as loosening of teeth. It is important to decide if periosteum is involved or not and if inferior alveolar nerve is involved.

The soft tissue margins are more important in determining survival rates than bony margins. Most cases rim resection suffices. Segmental resection is needed if:

a. Gross bone involvement in irradiated patients.
b. Medullary space is involved in non-irradiated patients (MRI scan shows medullary space involvement)
c. If there is less than 2 cm of bone after rim resection.

Segmental resection requires a fibular flap reconstruction.

Rim resection can involve alveolar margin or a rim of mandible on the lingual surface of the mandible. Retromolar trigone mass can be treated like an alveolar mass.

Maxillary alveolar masses may be treated by alveolectomy. But if it leaves a large oroantral fistula it has to be repaired with temporalis fascia. Extension to maxillary antrum and floor of nose requires more extensive surgery like maxillectomy through Weber-Ferguson's incision.

Describe malignancy of hard palate

Reverse smoking can cause squamous cell carcinoma. Otherwise the common tumor is adenoid cystic carcinoma. Other tumors can be adenocarcinoma, mucoepidermoid carcinoma, mucosal melanoma, Kaposi's tumor.

Differential diagnosis for palatal mass

1. Necrotizing sialometaplasia appears like a butterfly shaped ulcer in the palate and looks malignant. It is benign
2. Torus palatinus is a bony exotosis which occurs in the palate.

Surgery for squamous cell carcinoma of the hard palate depends on extent. Peroral excision can be done if tumor is small. If periosteum in involved bone is removed and if maxillary antrum is involved it will require maxillectomy. Large palatal defects can be closed by a dental obturator.

Verrucous carcinoma can be seen in the oral cavity.

Oral cavity mass rarely requires a mandibulotomy approach as opposed to oropharynx.

How will you treat lip cancer?

T_{1-2} N_0: Surgical excision/no neck dissection. If there is a positive margin either re-resection or radiotherapy can be tried.

T_{1-2} N_0 can also be treated with radiotherapy if residual tumor is seen after radiotherapy then surgery and reconstruction can be tried.

T_{3-4} N_0 and any TN_1–N_3: Surgery is preferred

In N_0: Excise primary. If there are no positive nodes only follow up is needed.
N1 excise primary + ipsilateral neck dissection
N_{2ab} N_3 excise primary + ipsilateral neck dissection
N_{2C} primary + bilateral neck dissection

If for some reason patient prefers RT than RT→following which if response is good only follow up.
If there is neck residue—neck dissection.
If there is primary site residue—salvage surgery.

Surgery and reconstruction in lip cancers:
Lower lip: Wedge excision
Loss of less than 1/3 lip: Primary closure.
1/3- 2/3 loss: Abbe-Estlander flap. A flap from the uninvolved lip is rotated to close the gap in the involved lip. The donor site is closed.
More than 2/3 lip loss: Karapandzic flap can also be used. Here tissue is rotated from the nasolabial fold and shifted medially and rotated to form the lower lip. Orbicularis oris muscle blood and nerve supply is retained and hence, there is a sensate flap.
For defects greater than 2/3 of the lip:

- Gillies fan flap
- Webster-Bernard reconstructions.

Gillies fan flap: Full thickness flap is made around the commissure extending on to the upper lip and nasolabial fold. This is rotated to close the defect in the lower lip.

Webster-Bernard flap, burrow's triangles are made from the edge of the lower lip excision, on both sides. The buccal mucosa from the base of the excised burrow's triangle is rotated inferiorly. The two flaps are advanced medially to close the lower lip defect. The triangles are closed.

Upper lip defects

1/3–2/3 defect:

- Reverse Karapandzic free flap.
- Abbe-Estlander flap.

In addition, upper lip defects between 1/3 to 2/3 can also be closed by perialar crescentic flap.

More than 2/3 of upper lip: A Burrow-Dieffenbach reconstruction can be done.

Defects of the commissure can be closed by Abbe-Estlander flaps.

What is the prognosis in lip cancer?

- 1 cm—94%, 5 year survival
- <2 cm—84%
- <4 cm—67%
- >4 cm—62%
- N_0—89%
- N_+ 61%.

Chapter 13

Oropharyngeal Mass

A 45-year-old male, mechanic by profession, presents with:

- Pain in the throat—2 years.
- Difficulty in opening his mouth—6 months.
- Wound/ulceration on left side of tongue—6 months.
- Difficulty in swallowing—6 months.
- Swelling in the neck left side—3 months.

HISTORY OF PRESENT ILLNESS

Pain in the throat is insidious in onset, gradually progressive continuous and mild to moderate in intensity.

Acute onset of severe throat pain is likely to be due to inflammatory lesions of the oral cavity, oropharynx or supraglottis. Throat irritation is also a common symptom.

Does the ulceration/wound on the tongue bleed spontaneously?

Yes, sometimes saliva is blood stained.

This is indicative of a neoplastic lesion.

Is there a foul smell emanating from it?

Yes, there is an odor.

Blood stained odorous masses may be due to local necrosis and secondary infection of a malignant mass.

Lymphoma's usually do not bleed or cause odor.

There are various instances when patient notices abnormalities on casual examination of his oral cavity and thinks it may be" cancer".

What are the structures mistaken for cancer by the patient?

Some structures are:

1. Lymphatic aggregates and vallate papillae.
2. Cysts in the tonsil.
3. Lingual thyroid swelling.

Single persistent ulcer lasting for more than 2–3 weeks should be viewed with suspicion and investigated

- Difficulty in opening his mouth is insidious in onset and gradually progressive.
- Normal opening of the jaw is 2–5 cm between upper and lower jaw.
- Acute onset of difficulty in opening his mouth can be due to tetanus and if so history of trauma should be asked for. In acute inflammatory lesions of the oral cavity, oropharynx and temperomandibular joint there may be difficulty in opening the mouth.

Do you have increased sensitivity to spicy foods?

No.
Inability to open mouth associated with sensitivity to spicy foods is seen in submucous fibrosis.

Difficulty in swallowing at first for solids; and now even liquids cannot be swallowed. There is drooling as he finds it difficult to swallow his saliva.

The trismus and pain both could be contributory factors for the difficulty in swallowing and drooling.

Do you have change in your voice?

Yes, there is some alteration in my voice because I cannot open my mouth and I also feel this ulcer in my mouth.

This can be a hot potato voice and is seen in oral, oropharyngeal and supraglottic lesions.

Do you have any difficulty in breathing?

No.
Airway obstruction is a late symptom in oral/oropharyngeal lesions.

Describe the swelling in your neck

The swelling in the neck was small about half this size and it has gradually become bigger.

Is it painful?

No.

Are there any other swellings in the neck?

No.

Where is this swelling exactly?

It is on the left side of the neck extending towards the middle of the neck.

Do you have any ear problem?

No.
Referred otalgia can occur due to glossopharyngeal and vagus nerves.
Otitis media with effusion can occur secondary to eustachian tube obstruction.

Do you have any impairment of tongue movements?

Yes.
This is usually seen due to infiltration of tongue muscles genioglossus. Muscle can propel malignant cells into the lymphatic system and spaces within tongue musculature.

Have you lost weight? Do you have evening rise of temperature or cough or loss of appetite?

No.
These are symptoms of tuberculosis.

PAST HISTORY

Do you have diabetes mellitus, hypertension, syphilis, dental problems such as sharp teeth?

No.
Diabetes mellitus and hypertension are comorbid conditions. Syphilis and sharp teeth are predisposing factor for oral and oropharyngeal malignancies.

Family History

No significant family history.

Personal History

Patient is a smoker and has been chewing betel nut for 20 years. He is not an alcoholic.

Smoking, betel nut chewing and alcoholism are predisposing factors for malignancies.

Human papilloma virus is a contributory factor in oropharyngeal malignancies, particularly tonsillar malignancies.

From the history, there is probably a malignant lesion because of the history, attendant voice change, trismus and neck mass.

The anatomic region may be the oropharynx, because patient points to the ulcer at back of the mouth and this is not easily visible to him.

Can it be tuberculosis?

There is no evening rise of temperature or cough; but pain in the throat, change in the voice and neck mass can occur in tuberculosis. Trismus is not a usual symptom. Ulcers are usually multiple in tuberculosis.

Examination

Examination of the oral cavity: Lips and angle of the mouth are normal.
Teeth (Dental formula):

1112	2122
2212	2122

Dental hygiene appears poor.

Nicotine staining of oral mucosa cheek and palate seen.
Alveolar margins are normal.
(Pull buccal mucosa outwards from gingivolabial sulcus).
Buccal mucosa and opening of parotid duct is normal. Some areas of buccal mucosa are nicotine-stained. Movement of the tongue is normal.
(Tip of tongue is placed over upper alveolus.)
This allows examination of the floor of mouth—normal.
Examination along the floor of the mouth from anterior to posterior end where it meets the tongue and anterior pillar are normal.
(use 2 tongue depressors)
Retromolar trigone—normal (coffin area).
Next examine tonsil, posterior pharyngeal wall, hard and soft palate.

Indirect laryngoscopy to view posterior third of tongue and rest of larynx.
Posterior rhinoscopy to visualize the upper aspect of the soft palate as well as lateral nasopharyngeal wall.

An ulceroproliferative mass is seen on the left posterior third of the tongue.
It is about 3 cm in largest dimension, extending to the midline up to the foramen cecum and posteriorly into the vallecula, but not filling it.
The epiglottis is free.
A clear margin of about 3 mm is seen between the mass in the vallecula and epiglottis. The rest of the larynx appears normal.
The arytenoids, aryepiglottic folds, ventricular bands and vocal cords are normal in structure.
Mobility of the vocal cord is normal. (No restrictions of vocal cord mobility).
Pooling of saliva is seen in both pyriform fossae.
Palpation reveals that the mass extends to the whole thickness of the tongue, extending up to the midline.
No induration is felt on the right posterior third of tongue or on the anterior two thirds of the tongue.
The mass is hard in consistency and the tongue is blood stained.
Bimanual palpation involves placing the forefinger of one hand over the tongue and the other hand in the neck posteriorly in the suprahyoid region.

Squamous cell carcinomas are hard. Lymphatic masses are rubbery.
Salivary gland tumors are firm and do not usually bleed and are not as hard as squamous cell carcinoma. They are more firm than lymphatic masses.

Examination of the neck: There is a level II single node 5 cm in greatest dimension, hard, mobile. There are no other masses in the neck and the laryngeal architecture is normal.

Specificity and sensitivity for staging neck nodes by palpation is 60–70%.
Neck node may undergo rapid increase in size and appear cystic due to degenerative necrosis and may be mistaken for a branchial cyst. Tonsillar malignances may also present with cystic secondaries.

INVESTIGATIONS

Computed tomography (CT) and Magnetic resonance imaging (MRI) to look for:

1. Size, site and extent of primary tumor.
2. Potential spread to parapharyngeal space, supraglottis, posterior pharyngeal wall up to nasopharynx and downwards to hypo-pharynx.
3. Bone invasion to maxilla and mandible.
4. Visualize ipsilateral and contralateral.
5. Neck nodes.

X-ray chest

1. Pulmonary diseases tuberculosis.
2. Pulmonary metastasis.
3. Synchronous primary in the chest.

Fine needle aspiration cytology (FNAC) of the neck node

Positron emission tomography (PET) scan for stage III and IV

Biopsy under general anesthesia

Human papilloma virus (HPV) testing by HPV in situ hybridization, p16 immunohistochemistry and HPV DNA polymerase chain reaction is done.

Using all three tests, it is possible to classify 98% of cases as HPV positive or HPV negative.

HPV positive tonsillar malignancies have better prognosis than HPV negative ones in squamous cell carcinoma.

Secondary in a cervical node points to a tonsillar malignancy if the primary is unknown.

Dental consultation is particularly important prior to radiotherapy.
Referral to speech pathologist to assess functional status.

Tests for comorbidities:

- Cardiovascular insufficiencies
- Diabetes mellitus
- Hypertension
- Smoking
- Alcoholism
- Chronic obstructive airway disease.

The most reliable index to predict outcome of treatment in head and neck malignancy is the adult comorbidity evaluation 27 (Ace 27). It is designed specifically for cancer \patients.

Staging: T_{4a} N_{2a} M_X Stage IVa

Tumor size is less than 4 cm; but inability to open mouth indicates spread to muscles of mastication (medial pterygoid). Hence, it is T_{4a}.

N_{2a} lpsi lateral node more than 3 cm, but less than 6 cm in greatest dimension.

Staging in oropharyngeal malignancies:

- T_1: 2 cm or less in greatest dimension
- T_2: More than 2 cm, but not greater than 4 cm in greatest dimension

- T_3: More than 4 cm or extension to lingual surface of epiglottis
- T_{4a}: invades larynx, extrinsic muscles of tongue, medial pterygoid, hard palate and mandible
- T_{4b}: Lateral pterygoid muscle, pterygoid plate, lateral nasopharynx, skull base or encasing carotid artery.
  If base tongue malignancy invades muscles, extends to lingual surface of epiglottis and vallecula, it does not mean larynx is involved.
- N_o
- N_1: Single node not more than 3 cm is greatest dimension
- N_2: Node more than 3 cm but less than 6 cm is greatest dimension lateral single
- N_{2a}: Single node more than 3 cm but less than 6 cm
- N_{2b}: Ipsilateral nodes more than 3 cm but less than 6 cm
- N_{2c}: Bilateral or contralateral nodes more than 3 cm but less than 6 cm
- N_3: Node more than 6 cm is greatest dimension
- Stage I: $T_1 N_0$
- Stage II: $T_2 N_0$
- Stage III: $T_3 N_0$, T_1, T_2N_1, T_3N_1
- Stage IVa: $T_{4a} N_0$, $T_{4a} N_1$, $T_1 N_2$, $T_2 N_2$, $T_3 N_2$, $T_{4a} N_2$
- Shape IVb: T_{4b} any NM_0, any TN_3
- Shape IVC: Any T, any N, M_1.

Heart system has modified this using patient variable and has come up with a staging more likely to predict outcome of disease.

- Stage I: $T_1T_2N_0N_1$
- Stage II: $T_3 N_0 N_1$, $T_4 N_0$; $T_1 T_2 N_2$
- Stage III: $T_1 T_2 N_3$, $T_3 N_2$: $T_4 N_1$
- Stage IV: $T_4 N_2$, N_3.

This system uses patient variables, tumor variables, treatment variables and comorbidities into consideration.

What are the histological variations of malignancies of oropharynx with percentage frequency of presentation?

1. Squamous cell carcinoma (75%).
2. Lymphoepithelioma is undifferentiated carcinoma and has high incidence of lymph node metastasis.
3. Lymphoma non-Hodgkin's laye bell type 223 together (25%).
4. Salivary gland tumors—most common adenoid cystic carcinoma (5%).

How is squamous cell carcinoma histologically graded?

1. Grade cannot be assessed.
2. G1 well differentiated.
3. G2 moderately differentiated.
4. G3 poorly differentiated.
5. G4 undifferentiated.

Can metastasis occur in oropharynx from distant sites?

Yes, breast, lung, prostate, stomach and kidney.
Soft tissue sarcoma is a rare tumor in the oropharynx.

What are the common sub-sites in which malignancies occur?

1. Faucial tonsil and pillar—50%.
2. Posterior third of tongue—40%.
3. Soft palate.
4. Posterior pharyngeal wall—10%.

So, how will you treat this patient?

Base you answer to this question on the format below.
If disease is: T_1 and T_2, N_0 nodes or T_1 N_1;

The two modalities can be either RT or surgery and neck dissection.
Modality 1: Following RT if there is residual disease then surgery has to be done. Otherwise follow up is enough.
Modality 2: Following surgery + neck dissection, if there is no adverse reaction then follow up is enough or RT can be given, but if margins are not free or if nodes show extracapsular spread then CTRT has to be given.

- T_2 N_1—RT/CT—good response—follow up
- Residual disease—salvage surgery
- T_3-T_{4a} N_1 Modality 1: Cancer treatment and research trust (CTRT)/residual disease—salvage surgery
- Modality 2: Surgery to primary + neck dissection
- If there is no adverse reaction then RT
- If there are no free margins or extracapsular spread in the nodes CTRT
- Modality 3: Induction CT followed by RT
- Primary + N_2 N_3: Modality 1 is RT/chemotherapy RT
- If there is residual primary then salvage surgery to primary or if neck nodes are present then neck dissection is needed
- Modality 2: Surgery for primary + neck dissection + CTRT

Neck dissection for oropharynx:

- N_0: Level I To IV clearance
- N_1: Modified radical neck dissection
- N_{2ab}: Modified radical neck dissection
- N_{2c}: Bilateral neck dissection.

So, this case falls under T_{4a} N_{2a} Mx Patient can be given RT/chemotherapy RT or primary surgery and neck dissection.

In the first scenario, chemotherapy or chemotherapy RT is given if there is a residual disease in the primary site, salvage surgery is required or if neck node is present, then neck dissection is necessary.

In the second scenario, if primary surgery and neck dissection is done, if there is residual disease then chemotherapy RT can be given.

In both scenarios, if no residual disease is seen, patient has to be followed up.

What are the surgical procedures available for oropharyngeal malignancies?

Transoral, transpharyngeal, transmanibular resection.
Transoral:
- No external incision
- Good for small T_1 exophytic tumors. It can be used for upper or anterior oropharynx
- Difficult to do if patient has trismus
- Exposure is limited
- Boyle Davis mouth gag can be used to expose some tumors
- Wound heals by primary or secondary intention
- CO_2 laser can be used for small tumors of tonsil or tongue base.

Transoral transcervical:
- Tongue and floor of the mouth is released in order to pull these structures below the mandible into the neck
- Affords better access to tongue base tumors
- Injury to the lingual artery and hypoglossal nerve can occur.

Transpharyngeal approach:
Can be through
- Suprahyoid pharyngotomy
- Lateral pharyngotomy.

Suprahyoid pharyngotomy:
- Only for small tumors. Large tumors cannot be visualized well
- Entry through vallecula
- Extension of incision is possible
- Functional outcome good.

Lateral pharygotomy:
- Entry posterior to thyroid ala on diseased side
- Larynx can be retracted to the opposite side once pharynx is opened.

Transmandibular approach:
- Mandibulotomy
- Mandibulectomy

Mandibulotomy:
- Lip splitting incision
- Mandibulotomy should be anterior to mental foramen, so that mental artery is not injured
- If artery is injured, ischemic necrosis is likely after radiotherapy
- Mandibulotomy incision can be straight or extra step deep V
- Mandibulotomy can only be done if mandibular periosteum is not involved
- An alternative to lip splitting incision is visor flap
- An intraoral incision in the gingivolabial sulcus elevates the check flap like a visor
- Visor flap can injure mental nerve and is not as good as lip splitting for exposure to posterior part of oropharynx

- The mandible can be swung and exposes the whole of the oropharynx and the primary can be resected
- If mandible is involved by disease, then mandibulectomy is needed
- If marrow space is involved, then 2 cm margin should be present beyond visible extent of tumor
- Depending on how much of the mandible is involved, whole of ramus, body and parasymphysis may have to be removed.

This patient needs a lip splitting incision, followed by a mandibulotomy; and once the mandible is swung, then the primary can be resected out. Since the mandible is not involved, it can be spared. N_{2a} neck requires a modified radical neck resection on the left side.

If surgery is the method of choice, if margins are clear, then radiotherapy has to be given.

If there are positive margins or extracapsular spread in the *node, then chemotherapy/RT should be started after 6 weeks.*

How will the wound heal? Do you need to reconstruct?

Healing can be by:

1. Primary intention
2. Secondary intention
3. Reconstruction
   - Local flaps
   - Regional flap
   - Microvascular free flap
   - Tubular free flap.

Tongue: If more than 30% of the tongue has to be reconstructed the best flap is sensate radial forearm flap or lateral arm flap.

The other flap that can be used is lateral thigh free flap.

If patient has co morbidities that prevent use of a microvascular free flap than a pectoralis major myocutaneous flap (regional flap) can be used. The problem with this flap is that it is bulky and hence cannot be remodeled in the oropharynx easily. Also because of the bulk dental rehabilitation becomes difficult. This flap also undergoes partial necrosis frequently.

Other regional flaps are latissimus dorsi myocutaneous flap, temporal and parietal flaps.

Tonsil and pharyngeal wall: If the defect is less than 4 cm it heals by secondary intention. Oro-palatal flap (local flap) if it is more than 4 cm. If larger than a radial forearm flap can be used.

Same with palatal defect. If small, it can heal by secondary infection or a local palatal flap. If large a radial forearm flap will be necessary.

In patients who have a number of comorbid conditions a microvascular free flap cannot be used. In such cases a pectoralis major myocutaneous flap is a better choice.

If mandible has to be reconstructed the best flap is fibula free flap.

If you decide on radiotherpy/chemoradiation how will you proceed?

The five modalities available are:

1. Induction chemotherapy/radiotherapy
   - Induction chemotherapy works only if 3 drugs are used.
   - This causes a problem for future chemo-irradiation as single doses of cisplatin cannot be given.
   - So, chemo-irradiation is better than induction chemotherapy followed by irradiation. Induction chemotherapy has an effect on distant metastasis but no effect on local control.
2. Irradiation
   - 64–74 Gy (2 Gy /fraction) 6 fractions/week/6 weeks
   - Hyperfractionation 81.6 Gy/7 weeks is given as 1.2 Gy/fraction/twice daily.
   - Hyperfractionation may have better control over local disease as compared to 2 Gy/when followed up after 5 years.
3. Postoperative radiotherapy
   - Primary 50–60 Gy (2 Gy/fraction)
   - Involved node 60–66 (2 Gy/fraction)
   - Uninvolved node 44–64 Gy.
   - More than 75 Gy conventional dose may lead to unacceptable normal tissue damage.
4. Chemo-irradiation:
   - 70 Gy to primary and gross adenopathy + cisplatin 100 mg/m^3 every 3 weeks—3 doses,
5. Intensity modulated radiotherapy works very well for oropharynx (IMRT):
   - In IMRT treatment, region is divided into hundreds of pencil beams; each of these beams targets a particular volume. A computer controls the amount of radiation delivered as the machine rotates around the patient.
   - Different tumor volumes to be irradiated such as primary, neck nodes, etc. are decided and organs to be protected are also mapped on a treatment CT scan.
   - Next, computer generates a treatment delivery plan which is evaluated by the radiation oncologist and then the patient's computer files are loaded into the delivery system.

   It can be delivered as:

   i. Simultaneous integrated boost: Uses different dose painting for different structures.
   5 doses/week.

   ii. Seqential IMRT uses different areas on different days.

   iii. Concomitant boost accelerated IMRT
   IMRT reduces dose to critical structure such as:
      1. Mandible
      2. Salivary glands

3. Spiral cord
4. Temporal bone
5. Auditory and optic structures.

How do you assess or predict programs for your patient?

Patient factor	*Tumors factor*	*Treatment factor*
Age	Site of origin	Resection margins
I	Maximum thickness	Time between surgery and radiotherapy
	Depth of invasion	
Comorbidity	Extracapsular spread of lymph node disease	

Cure is 0% if there is post-styloid space spread, prevertebral fascia involvement, carotid system involvement.

What is resectable/unresectable as opposed to moderately advanced/ very advanced?

Resectable refers to anatomical resectability which may not provide for improved prognosis. Both advanced and very advanced tumors can be resected but the prognosis is very poor for very advanced tumors.

Classify Neck Dissection

Neck dissection can be classified as comprehensive and selective.
Comprehensive neck dissection removes all nodes removed in classical radical neck dissection.
Whether sternomastoid muscle, accessory nerve and internal jugular vien is resected or not does not affect the term comprehensive neck dissection.
Selective neck dissection can be
1. Supraomohyoid I–III.
2. Extended Supraomohyoid I–IV.
3. Lateral neck dissection II–IV .
4. Anterior or central VI3
5. Posterolateral II–V.
6. Superior mediastinum VII.

In an N_0 neck in head and neck malignancies there is no drainage to nodes other than the designated nodes of drainage. So, selective neck dissection is for N_0 neck.

Chapter

14

Vocal Nodules

A 30-year-old woman presents with hoarseness of the voice—1 year.

HISTORY OF PRESENT ILLNESS

The voice has been hoarse for the past one year. It has been progressive and worse over the past 15 days. She had a respiratory infection which made her unable to use her voice. She says that she is a teacher by profession and has to strain a lot to speak.

Hoarseness is a coarse or rough sound which occurs when the free margins of the vocal cords are involved. Patients complain of hoarseness even when there is alteration in various other qualities of the voice. Dysphonia is an impairment of the voice or difficulty in speaking.

Other questions to ask about the voice are:

Is there breathiness? Yes, sometimes.

Breathiness is excess loss of air during phonation. If can be due to:

1. *Vocal fold paralysis.*
2. *Mass along free margin of cord.*
3. *Arthritis of cricoarytenoid joint.*
4. *Arytenoid dislocation.*
5. *Scarring of vibratory margin of cord.*
6. *Malignancy.*

Do you have vocal fatigue?

Yes, especially when I have to take many classes.

Fatigue indicates inability to maintain quality of voice over extended period of time.

It may be due to:

1. *Muscle fatigue caused by myasthenia gravis*
2. *Lamina propria fatigue may be due to dehydration, edema of vocal fold edges, overuse of voice*
3. *Abdominal or neck muscle fatigue.*

Is the dynamic range reduced?

Yes, dynamic range is reduced.
Each person has a voice range, i.e. the loudest and softest voice produced. This changes in

1. *Menopause.*
2. *Hormonal changes.*
3. *Aging.*
4. *Neurological problems.*
5. *Viral infection can cause superior laryngeal nerve paralysis reducing dynamic range.*

Is there diurnal variation of voice?

No.
Diurnal variation (voice worse in the evening) is seen in chronic laryngitis.

Is there pain during phonation?

No.
Pain during phonation can be due to

a. *Laryngitis*
b. *Cartilage infection*
c. *Singing or speech outside the dynamic range or misuse of voice.*

Did you have an upper respiratory tract infection/chronic cough?

Yes.
Upper respiratory tract infection can cause frequent clearing of throat and cough resulting in change of voice.

Is there any reason for dehydration like climate change/insufficient water intake?

No.
These can result in dehydration of vocal cords.

Has there been any inhalation of chemicals/noxious fumes?

No.
This causes edema of soft tissue of larynx resulting in hoarseness.

History of thyroid insufficiency like weight gain, loss of hair can be associated with hoarseness.

No.

Is there any cause of dysarthria?

No.
TM joint arthritis, dental disease can cause change in voice.

Is there history of previous surgery?

No.

Prior history of surgery can cause:

1. *Endotracheal intubation—trauma.*
2. *Thyroid surgery.*
3. *Anterior cervical spine surgery.*
4. *Thoracic surgery.*
5. *Abdominal surgery (recently) may prevent adequate voice production*
   2, 3 and 4 can cause recurrent laryngeal nerve paralysis.

Are you on any medication?

No.

Diuretics/vitamin C in large doses/antihistamines can have a dehydrating effect on the cords.

Hormonal therapy/hormone replacement therapy can also cause change in voice.

Are you a diabetic?

No.

Immunocompromised can develop fungal laryngitis.

Do you have nasal aspiration?/Do you have any central nervous system symptoms?

No.

Hoarseness can be a part of CNS involvement or lower cranial nerve involvement as in jugular bulb syndrome.

Do you have dysphagia or odynophagia?

No.

Some causes of hoarseness with dysphagia:

a. *Laryngopharyngeal reflux*
b. *Gastroesophageal reflux disease (GERD)*
c. *Mass involving oropharynx, laryngopharynx, esophagus.*
   a and b causes edema of larynx.
   c may involve recurrent laryngeal nerve.

Is there history of acid regurgitation or regurgitation of food?

No.

These occur in pharyngeal pouch and gastroesophageal reflux disease (GERD) and can cause hoarseness of voice.

Do you have stridor?

No.

Stridor is noise produced during respiration. Obstruction in the larynx produces inspiratory stridor. This is because in the larynx the airway is narrow during inspiration as the structures are sucked in. So any obstruction gets exaggerated at this stage of respiration. In the lungs, the negative pressure in the pleural space keeps the alveoli open during inspiration and it narrows during expiration. So, any obstruction exaggerates this narrowing and causes expiratory stridor. In the trachea, the rings neither narrow nor widen during any phase of respiration; hence stridor is biphasic.

Stridor with hoarseness can be seen in any obstruction lesion of the larynx and in subglottic malignancies where stridor is an important symptom along with hoarseness.

As the patient speaks the following can be assessed.

Is the voice rough?

No.
Asynchronous voice with sub-harmonics causes rough voice.

Is it breathy?

Yes.
Breathiness is due to leakage of air.

Is the voice weak?

No.
Asthenia can be due to large glottic chink and inability to produce adequate subglottic pressure.

Is the voice strained?

No.
Strained voice requires effort to produce.

What is Grade, Rough, Breathiness, Asthenia, Strain (GRBAS)?

This is a perceptual way of assessing voice and it correlates well with other assessments such as video stroboscopy, etc. It evaluates voice on quality. It has a bias because measurement is based on judgment.
GRBAS/auditory threshold assessment.
G: grade overall severity
R: rough
B: breathiness
A: asthenia
S: strained.

Is there any swelling in the neck?

No.

Hoarseness is a symptom of malignancy of glottis/supraglottis and can cause secondaries in the neck.
Tuberculosis can also cause cervical lymphadenitis and hoarseness of voice.

Past history:
- No history of evening rise of temperature loss of appetite, loss of weight and cough
- No history of syphilis, diabetes, hypertension.

Family history:
- Not significant.

Personal history:
- Not a smoker or alcoholic.

On examination:
- Oral cavity normal
- Oropharynx: normal/palatal movement normal
- Gag reflex present.

Indirect laryngoscopy: Posterior third of tongue normal. Vallecula, epiglottis, aryepiglottic fold, arytenoids normal. False cords normal. There are pin head sized white, opaque masses on the free margin of the vocal cords at the junction of the anterior one third with the posterior two thirds of the vocal cords. Both the masses are of the same size. It is sessile and does not extend to the superior or inferior surface of the cord. Anterior commissure appears normal. Vocal cord movements are normal. There is a small glottic chink anterior and posterior to the mass, which can be closed on effortful phonation.

Pyriform fossa normal. No other abnormalities seen.

Indirect laryngoscopy procedure: Use gauze to hold the tongue. The gauze should extend to the inferior surface of the tongue to prevent injury over the teeth when tongue is pulled forwards. The structures to be viewed are:
1. *Posterior third of tongue.*
2. *Epiglottis.*
3. *Vallecula.*
4. *Aryepiglottic folds.*
5. *Arytenoids.*
6. *False cords.*
7. *True cords.*
8. *Pyriform fossa.*

Next view the larynx asking the patient to breath deeply.
Lastly, patient should phonate ee-aah to look for cord mobility.
Failure to perform indirect layrngoscopy may be due to
a. *Exaggerated gag reflex*
b. *Overhanging epiglottis*
c. *Trismus due to any cause*
d. *Inability to extend tongue.*

In c) and d), tongue can be depressed with a tongue depressor.

What are the structures not seen on indirect laryngoscopy?

1. Anterior commissure.
2. Ventricle.
3. Infrahyoid epiglottis.
4. Subglottic region.
5. Apex of pyriform fossa.

Who discovered indirect laryngoscopy?

Manuel Garcia. He used a dental mirror and sunlight to view his own larynx.

How is the image seen on indirect laryngoscopy?

It gives good color and depth perception. Subtle changes due to vocal hermorhage can be visualized. Disadvantage is that only single phonatory sounds can be assessed, as tongue is fixed.

In cases of vocal cod paralysis, all cranial nerves should be examined to rule out polyneuropathy.

Examination of the neck

- Osseocartilaginous framework of the larynx and trachea is normal
- No neck nodes or swelling seen
- No thyroid enlargement
- Bocca's sign is negative.

If the laryngeal cartilages are moved against the vertebra, a grating sound is produced. This sound is absent if there is soft tissue interposed between larynx and vertebra as in postcricoid malignancy. Sound cannot be perceived if cricoid cartilage is damaged due to any reason.

- Examination of Nose and sinuses—Normal
- Ears—Normal
- Diagnosis—Vocal nodules.

What are vocal nodules?

It is a benign mucosal fold lesion.

What are the layers of the vocal fold?

Vocal cord has 5 layers:

1. Squamous epithelium (no mucous glands).
2. Superficial lamina propria.
3. Intermediate lamina propria.
4. Deep lamina propria.
5. Vocalis muscle.

How will you confirm your diagnosis?

1. 70 or 90 degrees telescope can be used to give a brighter and clearer picture. Image is more accurately magnified than flexible endoscope.

Here again phonation is limited to sustained vowel. Size of glottic chink appears larger, because tongue is pulled forwards and neck is extended.

2. Flexible endoscope
   Ability to view larynx during speech and singing. Glottic gap is more accurate as tongue is not pulled forwards. The light and magnification is inferior to rigid endoscope. Posterior part of larynx is not as well seen as in indirect laryngoscopy or telescope. There is a controversy over how to sterilize the endoscope.
3. Videolaryngoscopy
   Vocal cords vibrate rapidly at 256 times/sec. Images are retained on the retina for 0.2 sec. So every second only 5 images are visualized. In stroboscopy the image is formed by viewing different points of phonation on consequent phonatory cycles, so that it looks like a continuous wave and a simple wave motion. But what you really view are different cycles at points consequent to one another. The slow motion effect occurs because the stroboscope light and vocal cord vibration are desynchronized at about 2 Hz. If vocal cord movement and stroboscope are synchronized, the vocal cords will appear immobile.
   Instruments needed for videolaryngostroboscopy are:
   i. Stroboscopic light source
   ii. Endoscope
   iii. Microphone
   iv. Video camera
   v. Recording device
   vi. Video monitor.
   Recording is done when patient performs various tasks like speaking, singing in low, normal and high pitches. The factors of the vibratory cycle to be looked for are
   i. Symmetry—symmetry is present if the glottic margins are normal.
   ii. Periodicity
   iii. Amplitude of vibration
   iv. Shape and contour of glottic margin
   v. Glottal closure
      a. Complete
      b. Incomplete with anterior, middle on posterior chinks
         Hour glass chink is seen in vocal nodule.
      - In vocal nodule:
        Waves are symmetric
        Reduced amplitude of vibration
        Periodicity is normal
        Hour glass closure is seen.
      - In vocal polyp:
        Since it is unilateral, wave is asymmetric.
        Variable periodicity.
        Mucosal wave is absent if mass is large, but intact if mass is broad based.

In unilateral lesions wave is intact on the normal side.

Videolaryngostroboscopy is not as good as high speed photography or high speed digital video because videolarygostroboscopy studies many cycles.

4. Electroglottography: Two electrodes are placed on either side of the thyroid lamina and the impedance studied. If cords are touching current flows through. EGG wave is studied. If there is cord palsy, this test cannot be done. If there is severe hoarseness, it cannot be done as laryngeal irritation can occur.
5. Photoglottography: Light passes through the glottis depending on how open it is, so this can study the symmetry of the opening and closing parts of the open phase and calculate the open quotient.
6. Ultrasound glottography: If glottis is open, no signal is got as air does not transmit the ultrasound.
7. High speed photography: Photograph has to be taken with an indirect laryngoscopy mirror. So patient has to cooperate. High speed imaging uses endoscopes to record images.
8. Acoustic voice measurement can be made with commercially available voice analysers like Dr Speech. Quality of voice such as jitter and shimmer can be studied. Jitter is variation in pitch. Shimmer is variation in intensity.
   All investigations need not be done in all cases. Electromyography is more relevant for cord paralysis.

What are the other mucosal lesions?

1. Polyp.
2. Laryngeal varices/ectasia.
3. Vocal sulcus.
4. Intracordal cyst.

How are nodules caused?

Mid membranous vocal fold experiences maximal strain. This repeated collision causes localized vascular congestion and edema. Eventually, hyalinization of Reinke's space and thickening of epithelium over it occurs.

How does it differ from a polyp?

Polyp is usually unilateral and pedunculated. It occurs after acute voice abuse or anticoagulant intake or endotracheal intubation. It is due to breakage of capillaries in Reinke's space and extravasation of blood, local edema and hyalinization of stroma.

What are cysts/vocal sulcus?

- Cysts are subepidermal epithelial lined sacs. It can be rupture and become a sulcus
- Vocal sulcus: Type I extends to superficial lamina propria alone
- Type II extends beyond vocal ligament

- Type III: Deep focal indentation resembling a pit
- Videostrobosocpy shows asymmetric amplitude of vibration, loss of mucosal wave.

What is the treatment for mucosal lesions?

Prevention is the best treatment. Avoiding vocal trauma, having a well hydrated larynx, avoiding allergens, GERD, laryngopharyngeal reflux. Speech therapy is also effective is avoiding these lesions.

What is the surgical treatment?

- Microlaryngeal surgery
- Position: Neck flexed and extension at atlantoaxial joint
- Microlaryngeal surgery allows binocular vision, magnification and ability to use cold steel/laser/powered instruments
- Laser is good for vascular lesions. Microdebrider is good for papilloma's as it eliminates spread of virus through laser plume if laser is used. Nodule is held with micro forceps and micro-scissor is used to cut the nodule out preserving as much mucosa as is possible. Both nodules can be removed at the same time.

What is Reinke's oedema?

This is edema of the vocal folds seen in smokers and patients with GERD.

- Grade I: Marginal edge edema
- Grade II: Sessile swelling
- Grade III: Large bag like swelling filled with fluid.
- Grade IV: Partially obstructive lesion
- Incision is made on superior surface of cord laterally, mucosa elevated and contents of Reinke's space aspirated.

Chapter 15

Left Vocal Cord Paralysis

A 45-year-old man presents with dysphonia 3 months.
Breathiness of voice—3 months.

HISTORY OF PRESENT ILLNESS

He says that he noticed about 3 months ago that he could not produce a voice of sufficient intensity. He has been to a general practitioner who gave him medicines but he continues to have the same problem. He says that he has to work hard to produce a voice which is not as loud as it was before. Other than everyday speech, he does not use his voice for anything else because it is an effort to speak. He also has voice fatigue. His dynamic range has reduced as he cannot produce a loud voice. There is no pain during phonation.

- No history of respiratory tract infection.

Viral infections can cause a weak voice due to superior laryngeal nerve paralysis

- No cough or blood stained sputum.

The first symptom of bronchogenic carcinoma can be a weak voice

- No nasal symptoms
- Nasopharyngeal carcinoma can cause lower cranial nerve palsies
- No history of dysphagia/weight loss.

Esophageal malignancies can causes weak voice due to recurrent laryngeal nerve paralysis

- No accidental or iatrogenic trauma
- No history of loss of consciousness/altered speech/gait/aspiration

All suggestive of base of brain involvement/jugular foramen syndrome

- Grade, roughness, breathiness, asthemia, strain (GRBAS)
- Voice is asthenic and breathy.

From the history, it could be a benign mucosal lesion/benign swelling/cord paralysis

- Not malignant as there is no hoarseness.

On Examination

- Oral cavity normal
- Oropharynx: no palatal paralysis/gag reflex +/no lymphoid tissue hypertrophy
- No postnasal drip
- Indirect laryngoscopy
- Posterior third of tongue normal.
- Vallecula, epiglottis normal.
- Aryepiglottic fold on the left side appears to be drawn inwards, as compared to the right side
- On phonation: The left vocal cord lies in the cadaveric position. The right vocal cord is in the paramedian position. There is no bowing of the vocal cords
- The left cord appears shorter than the right and is at a lower level
- *Contraction of the normal cricothyroid muscle rotates the posterior commissure towards the inactive side and so the cord appears shorter and rima glottidis appears oblique*
- *The arytenoids cartilage is normal on both sides*
- *The arytenoids can be drawn forwards due to the unopposed action of the lateral cricoarytenoid muscle which may be less involved, whereas the posterior cricoarytenoid may be totally paralyzed*
- *The cricothyroid muscle is essential to maintain cord in paramedian position*
- No pooling of saliva in the pyriform fossa; no odema of arytenoids
- *Both indicate hold up of food*
- Anterior and posterior rhinoscopy—normal.
- Ears normal
- Cardiovascular system (CVS): No abnormality detected (NAD)
- Respiratory system (RS) No abnormality detected (NAD)
- *Left vocal cord can be paralysed due to left ventricular hypertrophy/ patent ductus arteriosis.*

Diagnosis: Left vocal cord paralysis? Idiopathic.

Why do you say idiopathic/what are the causes of recurrent laryngeal nerve paralysis?

1. Iatrogenic trauma as in:
   - Thyroid surgery
   - Anterior cervical spine surgery
   - Thoracic surgery

   Nerve may be:
   a. Transected
   b. Crushed
   c. Injured due to traction
   d. Included in ligature
   e. Thermal injury (cautery).

2. Non-iatrogenic trauma (accidental)
3. Neurological diseases:
   a. Multiple sclerosis
   b. Amyotrophic lateral sclerosis
   c. Myasthenia gravis
   d. Guillain Barre's syndrome
   e. Parkinson's disease
   f. Cerebrovascular accidents
   g. Recurrent laryngeal nerve neuropathy in diabetes.
4. Tumor infiltration or compression
5. Infection
6. Collagen vascular disease
7. Idiopathic.

Do you think the superior laryngeal nerve is involved?

No, there is no bowing of the cord.

What are the causes of superior laryngeal nerve involvement?

Thyroidectomy/viral infections/compensatory mechanism in muscle tension dysphonia.

What are signs and symptoms of superior laryngeal nerve paralysis?

Lowered pitch of voice, vocal fatigue, breathiness, loss of upper range of voice.

Indirect laryngoscopy may appear normal or show a bowed vocal fold. Vocal fold may be slightly arched, glottic closure may be incomplete.

How will you investigate?

- All tests as in chapter 14/electromyography
- CT scan of neck and chest
- Upper GI endoscopy/bronchoscopy.

How do you classify nerve paralysis?

Sunderland's classification:
- First degree—neuropraxia
- Second degree—Wallerain degeneration distal to injury axonotmesis
  No synkinesis occurs as endoneural sheath is intact
- Third degree—endoneural scarring, misdirected regeneration
- Fourth degree—scarring can block regeneration
- Fifth degree—transaction (neuromesis).

Why is the left recurrent laryngeal nerve commonly involved?

It has a longer course. It passes inferior and posterior to the aortic arch and reverses its course to continue into the neck.

Right recurrent laryngeal nerve winds round the subclavian artery.

What is non-recurrent laryngeal nerve?

Right nerve is non-recurrent in 0.5% people.

What is electromyography?

Interior of the muscle cell is negative and exterior is positively charged. So, there is a resting membrane potential. Appropriate stimuli such as needle electrodes inserted into the muscle, causes an action potential.

Laryngeal muscle fibers are a combination of:

Type I: Sustained low intensity contraction (aerobic)

Type II A: Short bursts of high activity (anaerobic)

Type II B: Intermediate activity.

Electromyograph:

1. Insertional activity when eletrode is inserted.
2. Spontaneous activity.

   Normal muscle shows no activity, while denervated muscle shows spontaneous activity indicating degeneration.

   This is seen usually as a normal upward spike followed by a downward spike (biphasic).
3. During denervation there are no wave forms.

   During reinnervation there are small amplitude waves. During reinnervation, as all nerve fibers do not regenerate, more motor plates are innervated by a small number of nerves; so, there is polyphasic myopotential.

What are the chances of recovery?

Synkinesis causes non-selective innervation of adductor and abductor muscles, so that the action cancels itself out. So, functionally there is no phonation possible.

Synkinesis is of 4 types:

Type I: Favorable synkinesis resulting in no movement of vocal cord.

Type II: Spastic vocal fold which twitches without control.

Type III: Tonic adduction of cords may cause airway obstruction (more lateral cricoarytenoid muscle fibers are innervated).

Type IV: Tonic abduction resulting in a weak voice (more posterior cricoarytenoid muscle fibers are innervated).

What are treatment modalities available for cord palsies?

1. Speech therapy
2. Injection laryngoplasty:
   a. Teflon (polytetrafluoroethylene causes granulomatous reaction)
   b. Absorbable gelatine powder (gets absorbed)
   c. Fat gets absorbed in 3–4 months
   d. Collagen
   e. Dermal collagen
   f. Hydroxypatite

3. **Medialiazation:** Delay for at least one year after palsy.
   Medial displacement of cord with an implant (Type I thyroplasty). Implants can be silastic, hydroxyapatite, Gortex. Posterior gap is closed by aryteriod adduction. Sometimes arytenoid can be fixed in the midline position.
4. **Muscle reinnervation:** Reinnervation fails because laryngeal muscles are Type II predominantly, and strap muscles are Type I. The distribution of end plates in both types is different. So reinnervation is difficult. Omohyoid muscle has been placed in posterior cricoarytenoid and lateral cricoarytenoid muscles; but results are not very good.
5. **Vocal cord pace maker:** Laryngeal pacemaker has been tried. One problem is, muscle has to be stimulated in a coordinated manner. For example, if paralyzed side abducts and normal side adducts, it is of no use.

How does compensation occur in recurrent laryngeal nerve paralysis?

Compensation can only happen if both cords are in the same level. If cricothyroid muscle is normal, then in higher pitches the paralyzed cord can come to paramedian position by stretching, and if normal opposite cord acts to overreach then compensation happens. All this fails if cords are not in the same level.

What will you do for bilateral vocal cord paralysis?

Tracheostomy may be required immediately.

Endoscopic laser (CO_2) cordotomy and arytenoidectomy with or without vocal cord lateralization can be done.

What is muscle tension dysphonia?

There is excessive muscular effort during phonation. It may occur due to vocal cord pathology such as cord palsy where extra effort is needed to narrow the rima glottidis. Sometimes, it happens even in normal larynges. There is hyperadduction of vocal cords and anterior and posterior compression of glottis. Identifying the cause and speech therapy helps.

What are the common causes of voice alteration?

1. Pulmonary pathology like asthma/emphysema
2. Laryngeal lubrication deficit due to drugs or otherwise/alcohol
3. Oral contraceptives
4. Tobacco/GERD
5. Endocrine disorders like hypothyroidism.

Chapter 16

Supraglottic Carcinoma

A 55-year-old man agriculturist by profession presents with swelling right side of neck 1 month.

He also has change in voice—2 months.

HISTORY OF PRESENTING ILLNESS

The man presented with a swelling right side of neck which was initially small (size of a grape) which increased to size of a small lemon. It is painless and gives him no problems. He also has change in voice 2 months duration. He has not taken any treatment for this as it is painless and the roughness does not bother him.

- He reports no increased effort during phonation. He also does not notice any change in dynamic range as he does not use his voice professionally
- No history of vocal fatigue or breathiness of voice
- No history of dysphagia
- No history of stridor
  (*All questions as in chapter 18*)
- He is a smoker and alcoholic (smokes 2 packets of beedies/day and has 60 mL of country made liquor everyday.
  (*Beedi is tobacco shavings wrapped in tendu leaf*)

Alcohol promotes carcinogenesis through acetaldehyde exposure, malnutrition and dissecation of mucosa. Tobacco acts via polycyclic aromatic hydrocarbons like benzopyrine whose products bind to DNA and RNA.

Do people not exposed to tobacco and alcohol get cancer larynx?

- Yes, but it occurs almost 10 years later and it is mostly glottic
- 75% of head and neck cancers are caused by alcohol/tobacco
- 25% are caused by Human papillomma virus
- HPV E_6 and E_7 disrupt P_{53} and PRb
- HPV 16, 21, 8 associated with oropharyngeal cancer
- HPV_{11} genome causes recurrent papillomatosis.

What is the genetic process leading to head and neck cancers?

There can be chromosomal loss, chromosomal gain or amplification.

1. Hyperplasia loss of chromosome 9_p12. This encodes P_{16} (a tumor suppressor gene) which inhibits cell cycle from G1 check point to S phase by inhibiting phosphorylation of PRb.
2. Dysplasia—loss of 3_p21 and 17_p 13 (Contains P_{53}).
   P_{53} plays a role in DNA repair, cell cycle progression and apoptosis.
3. Carcinoma in situ—loss of 13_q21 and 14_q 32 and amplification of 11_q3.
   PRb is contained in 13_q21 and controls cell cycle progression and apoptosis.
4. Invasive carcinoma has specific allelic loss—$6_p8_p4_p27$ and 10_q12.
   Subsequently, there is loss of $3_{p,}5_{q,}8_{p,}9_{p,}13_{p,}$ 18q and 21q.
   3p and 9p loss has 3.8 fold increase risk for progression to cancer. Additional loss of 4p, 8p, 11q and 17p increases the risk 33 fold.

What does this tell us?

We can be more aggressive in treating patients with 3_p and 9_p loss. If these patterns are known then wild P_{53} immunomodulatory genes can be injected into dysplastic and cancerous cells using a recombinant adenovirus.

P_{53} and immunemodulatory genes such as granulocyte macrophage colony stimulating factor (GM-CSF) and B7-1 genes using a recombinant adenovirus induces cell apoptosis.

Genes can also be silenced by DNA hypermethylation and chromatin remodeling.

Epidermal growth factor receptor (EGFR) is a transmembrane tyrosine kinase receptor which plays a role in cell survival and proliferation. Over expression of EGFR is seen with early disease progression, poor survival and resistance to chemotherapy. Blocking EGFR signal transduction pathway is a potential anticancer treatment. Cetuximab is an anti-EGFR antibody and can be given with CTRT.

EGFR can also be targeted using TKIs which target EGFR's intracellular machinery. These are less specific as they work on the downstream mechanism. It can be used in recurrent and metastatic tumors when used with CT. Sometimes anti-EGFR factors and TKIs can be used together.

Tumor environment is altered by matrix metalloproteinases which cause basement membrane disruption, stroma and blood vessel penetration and metastasis. There is over expression of matrix metalloproteinases in head and neck cancers. This is over expression can predict nodal and distant metastasis.

Vascular endothelial growth factor plays a role in angiogenesis, some VEGF inhibitors are Bevacizumab.

To alter systemic environment, immune function is altered such as lack of delayed hypersensitivity reaction. There is expression of immunosuppressive mediators, altered tumor antigen processing and presentation and impaired dendritic cell and lymphocyte function.

IL_4, IL_6, IL_8, IL_{10} and prostaglandin secretion is high. These are immune suppressor cytokines. TH_2 is secreted in excess of TH_1 (increases response against tumor) which can suppress responses against tumors. Dendrite cells are antigen presenting cells and their secretion is suppressed.

Immune response can be altered by adding IL2 and IL12 to the CTRT regime.

Thymic hormone also regulates immune response by modulating monocyte activity.

Some fungus like schizophyllum commune ferris and low virulence *Steptococcus pyogenes* are antineoplastic.

Vaccine against HPV is useful.

- No family history of similar complaints.
- General examination: as for all cases.

Generalized lymphadenopathy indicates at least 3 groups of lymph node enlargement.

On Examination

Oral cavity mucosa of cheek, gingiva show pigmentation which is blackish in color.

Dental formula	2211	2123
	2211	0122

Dental hygiene is poor.

Important, as poor dental hygiene can cause osteoradionecrosis of bones during irradiation.

Indirect laryngoscopy: Posterior third of tongue normal. There is an ulceroproliferative mass involving the right aryepiglottic fold extending to the right margin of the epiglottis and to the arytenoid posteriorly. Mass also involves the lateral surface of aryepiglottic fold. Epiglottic tip is seen, left margin and rest of epiglottis appears normal. Right ventricular band architecture is lost, the phonatory edge of the right vocal cord is seen only in the posterior third. Anterior two thirds of the right cord area: only mass is seen. Anterior commissure is involved by mass.

Left vocal cord, ventricular band left aryepiglottic fold, left arytenoid are normal. Both pyriform fossa free. No pooling of saliva in the pyriform fossa.

On phonation right cord mobility is restricted, left cord mobility is normal. No glottic chink is seen as mass covers rima glottidis on phonation.

Examination of the neck

Laryngeal framework is normal. No tenderness on palpation of thyroid or other cartilages.

Bocca's sign negative.

The swelling on the right side of neck is 3 cm in greatest dimension. Skin over the swelling normal, swelling is non-pulsatile. It is situated at the level of hyoid and thyroid cartilages along the anterior border of sternomastoid muscle.

On palpation it is hard in consistency, mobile vertically and horizontally.

Restricted vertical mobility may indicate fixation to carotid sheath or mass arising from carotid sheath.

No other palpable nodes in the neck.

- Ears—NAD
- Nose—NAD

Diagnosis: Malignancy of the supraglottis extending to glottis (transglottic) with secondaries in the neck.

Stage: T_3 N_1 M_x stage III.

Do you feel it could be tuberculosis?

Absence of pain: Tuberculosis laryngitis is painful due to cartilage involvement. Nodes in this case are hard and not matted.

What is transglottic tumor?

Cancer involving both glottis and supraglottis with vocal cord fixation. It probably arises from the laryngeal ventricle. They may involve laryngeal framework. It involves paraglottic space.

Tumors become transglottic in four ways:

i. By crossing ventricle in a vertical plane
ii. Through the anterior commissure
iii. Spread through the paraglottic space
iv. Spread along arytenoids cartilage posterior to ventricle.

What are the symptoms of supraglottic tumors?

Normal symptoms are globus, foreign body sensation, hot potato voice, paresthesia, hoarseness if it extends to glottis. Lesion may be asymptomatic till nodes appear.

How do you stage supraglottic tumors?

- Tx: Tumor not assessed
- T_0: No evidence of primary tumor
- Tis: carcinoma in situ
- T_1 tumor limited to one subsite of supraglottis with normal cord mobility
- T_2 tumor involves more than one subsite of supraglottis or glottis or region outside supraglottis/base tongue, vallecula, medial wall of pyriform fossa without fixation of larynx
- T_3 tumor limited to larynx with fixed cord and/or invades any of the following: postcricoid region, pre-epiglottic space, paraglottic space/and or inner cortex of thyroid cartilage
- T_{4a} Moderately advanced local disease
- Tumor invades thyroid cartilage and/or invades tissues beyond larynx (trachea, soft tissue of neck, deep muscles of tongue, strap muscles, thyroid or esophagus)

- T_{4b} very advanced local disease
- Spread to prevertebral region, mediastinum, encases carotid artery.

What are the subsites of the supraglottis?

- Epiglottis, tip, lingual and laryngeal surfaces
- Aryepiglottic fold
- Arytenoids
- Ventricle
- False cords.

What is the lower limit of supraglottis?

It is a horizontal line passing through the apex of the ventricle. Anatomically it is the superior arcuate line.

How do you stage supraglottic tumors?

- Stage 0 T_{1s}, N_0 M_0
- Stage I T_1 N_0 M_0
- Stage II T_2 N_0 M_0
- Stage III T_3 N_0 M_0
  $T_{1,}$ T_2, T_3, N_1 M_0
- Stage IVA T_{4a} N_0 M_0
  T_{4a} N1 M_0
  T_1 T_2 T_3 T_{4a} N_2 M_0
- Stage IVB T_{4b} Any N M_0
  Any T N_3 M_0
- Stage IVC Any T Any N M_1.

How do supraglottic tumors spread?

It depends on the site:
Suprahyoid epiglottis spreads to base of tongue, vallecula, aryepiglottic fold. Infrahyoid epiglottis spreads to preepiglottic space and then to paraglottic space or to thyrohyoid membrane. It can also spread to anterior commissure and glottis.
Ventricular band:
Quadrangular membrane limits inferior spread and is the basis for supraglottic laryngectomy.

Aryepiglottic fold and arytenoids spread to pyriform fossa and also to neck nodes. It is called marginal zone and behaves like hypopharyngeal tumors. Tumors are aggressive.

What are the natural barriers to tumor spread?

i. The overlying perichondrium of thyroid and cricoid cartilages
ii. Ventricle
iii. Conus elasticus

iv. Quadrangular membrane
v. Thyrohyoid membrane
vi. Hyoepiglottic ligament.

What does not resist tumor spread?

1. Anterior commissure/subglottic wedge. It was believed that anterior commissure tendon (Broyle's ligament) resists tumor spread; but once it is involved, the tumor spreads vertically in an upward and downward direction. This also happens because there is no inner perichondrium below the attachment of Broyle's ligament in an area called subglottic wedge.
2. Thyrohyoid membrane where the vascular structures pierce, it is a performed pathway.
3. Fenestrations in the epiglottis.
4. Preepiglottic space.
5. Paraglottic space.

What is pre-epiglottic space?

- The superior boundary is hypoepiglottic ligament
- The anterior boundary is thyroid cartilage and thyrohyoid membrane
- The posterior boundary is epiglottis and thyroepiglottic ligament
- Contents of preepiglottic space: fat, blood and lymphatic vessels.

What is paraglottic space?

It is a potential space and forms a horseshoe shaped space around the larynx. It allows cephalocaudal spread of tumor.
Lateral boundary: Thyroid cartilage anteriorly and mucosa overlying pyriform fossa posteriorly.

Superiorly and medially quadrangular membrane and inferiorly the conus elasticus. Paraglottic space involvement not only allows spread from supraglottis to glottis and also to subglottis and soft tissues of neck.

How will you investigate this patient?

1. Fiberoptic laryngoscopy
2. 70° or 90° telescope
3. X-ray neck anteroposterior and lateral views
4. X-ray chest:
   a. To rule out concomitant tuberculosis
   b. To rule out synchronous primary in the lung
   c. To look for mediastinal widening
   d. To rule out emphysematous changes
5. CT scan of neck to visualize:
   a. Preepiglottic space
   b. Paralgottic space

   c. Thyroid gland invasion
   d. Cartilage invasion
   e. Neck node evaluation
      (clinical examination is 25–50% false negative)
   f. Tumor volume
   g. PET/CT allows detection of subtle changes by altered metabolic activity and may change course of treatment
   h. Extralaryngeal spread
6. Direct laryngoscopy and biopsy
7. Upper GI endoscopy/barium swallow
8. ? Pan endoscopy
   For: Endoscopy may discover early lesions
   Against: CT/MRI does a better job
9. Work up for metastasis/lung/liver
10. Oxidized flavin mononucleotide is present in normal cells and emits green fluorescence when exposed to blue light. Cancer cells have significantly lower fluorescence.
11. Dental opinion
12. Speech pathologist and nutritionist.

After the investigations will the staging change?

Yes, it can. This is known as Will Roger's phenomenon.

What are the fallacies of staging in supraglottic tumors?

A large supraglottic of 3 cm is still T_1, whereas in the glottis it becomes T_3 and hence when prognosis is given it goes against glottis. Supraglottis T_3 denotes fixed cord/pyriform fossa involvement/postcricoid involvement/ preepiglottic space involvement. All these do not have the same prognosis. Each of these could have different prognosis.

In N staging only size and member of nodes are taken into account, whereas extracapsular spread and nodes which are palpable but do not contain cancer are not dealt with.

To a large number of staging, like IV, a, b, c group staging, the numbers are very small in each group and so accurate prognosis cannot be predicted.

What is TANIS?

This is an improved staging system. It combines the integers of T and N.

- $T_1 N_0$—Tanis 1
- $T_2 N_2$—Tanis 4

So group Tanis is:

- 1-3—Tanis 1
- 4—Tanis 2
- 5-7—Tanis 3

But problem here is T and N are considered same.

- T_2 No—Tanis 2
- T_1N_1—Tanis 2

} Whereas these do not have the same survival rate.

- Tanis does not include M.

How will you Treat this Patient?

Patient can be treated by surgery:
Total laryngectomy with thyroidectomy and bilateral neck dissection (functional on the left side)
If margins are clear and if there is no extracapsular spread in the node, patient can be given postoperative RT
If there is extracapsular spread or positive margins, CTRT.

A second line can be CTRT.
70 Gy conventional fractionation to primary and involved neck.
+44 - 64 Gy for uninvolved neck.

+

Cisplatin 100 mg/m^2 x 3 doses every 3 weeks.
If primary and neck show good response, observe.
If primary is residual, do total laryngectomy + thyroidectomy + bilateral neck dissection.
If neck shows residual disease and there is no residual primary, do neck dissection.

Do you want to try altered fractionation?

If CT is given along with RT, conventional fractionation causes less toxicity.

What will you do for smaller supraglottic tumors?

In $T_1T_2N_0$, any of the following three modalities can be tried.

1. Endoscopic resection
2. Open supraglottic laryngectomy
3. RT

In T_1 T_2 T_3 N_1 any of the following two modalities can be tried.

1. CTRT
2. Supraglothic laryngectomy (if no contraindication + bilateral neck dissection)

   In T_3 N_2 N_3: CTRT or surgery.

   In T_{4A} N_0 to N_3: Surgery; if refused, CTRT.
   In T_1T_2: Organ preservation.
   In T_3T_4: Organ preservation if cartilage is not involved. Through and through cartilage invasion requires surgery. In minor cartilage invasions, CTRT can be given.

What are the contraindications for supraglottic laryngectomy?

1. Should not involve ventricle.
2. Not extend excessively to posterior paraglottic space.

3. Preferably not involve supra hyoid epiglottis. If it is involved, the clearance in the tongue region will be poor.
4. Arytenoids should not be fixed.

What is supraglottic laryngectomy?

- Supraglottis is removed with cuts through vallecula, aryepiglottic folds and ventricle, upper half of thyroid cartilage and epiglottis. It can be done endoscopically or by open method.
- Endoscopy removes tumor piecemeal.
- Open method causes:
  - More aspiration
  - Glottic incompetence
  - Inadequate motor function
  - Loss of sensory innervation.

Complications of supraglottic laryngectomy are aspiration and deglutition problems.

Should patient stop smoking now, will it help?

Even after diagnosis, patient should stop smoking to prevent recurrence and field cancerization.

Describe endoscopic resection for supraglottis?

Since supraglottis is oval in cross section, an oval distending laryngoscope is needed. Instrument to apply vascular ligation clips is needed. If possible, enbloc resection should be attempted; because removing piecemeal is against oncological belief held as of now.

Chapter 17

Glottic Cancer

A 55-year-old laborer presents with hoarseness of voice 3 months.

HISTORY OF PRESENT ILLNESS

His voice has been hoarse for the past 3 months. It started as mild hoarseness which has been progressing to reach the present state. Now, he finds it difficult to raise his voice (*lowered dynamic range*). He finds it harder to produce the voice (*possibly cords are not meeting in the midline*).

He has been to a doctor who treated him with medicines but the hoarseness kept getting worse.

No other positive history.
(*Ask all questions as in chapter 14*)

He is a smoker and an alcoholic. He smokes about 3–3½ packets of beedi everyday and consumes alcohol about 3–4 days a week (60 mL).

General examination as in all cases.

On Examination

Oral cavity shows pigmentation of buccal mucosa.
Dental hygiene is poor and patient is almost edentulous.
2210 1121
2210 0122

Oropharynx: No loss of gag reflex/palate normal.

Indirect laryngoscopy: Posterior one-third of tongue is normal. Vallecula, epiglottis normal. Aryepiglottic folds, aryteniod and ventricular bands normal. There is an ulceroproliferative mass involving the free margin and superior surface of the left vocal cord in its anterior two-third. This mass extends to anterior commissure and mass is seen on the anterior one-third of the right vocal cord along the free margin and on 2 mm of the superior surface. The mass over the left cord and anterior commissure projects on to the rima glottidis but does not occlude it fully. The mass on the right cord is not as prominent as on the left. The posterior one-third of the left cord and posterior two-third of the right cord are normal. The arytenoids are normal. No pooling of saliva in the pyriform fossa. No abnormality seen in the pyriform fossa.

On phonation the right cord is mobile and the left cord shows restricted mobility. Subglottic area not seen.

Examination of the neck—NAD

Examination of the ear and nose—NAD

Diagnosis: Malignancy of glottis

$T_2 N_0 M_0$ stage II.

What is T Staging of glottis?

- T_1 Tumor limited to one vocal cord may involve anterior and posterior commissure with normal mobility.
- T_{1a} Tumor involves one cord.
- $T1_b$ Tumor involves both cords.
- T_2 Tumor extends to supraglottis or subglottis and/or restricted mobility.
- T_3 Tumor limited to larynx with vocal cord fixation and/or invasion of paraglottic space and/or inner cortex of thyroid cartilage.
- T_{4a} Moderately advanced local disease. Tumor involves outer cortex of thyroid cartilage and/or involves tissues beyond larynx, e.g. trachea, soft tissues of neck including deep extrinsic muscles of tongue, strap muscles/ thyroid gland and/or esophagus.
- T_{4b} very advanced local disease
  1. Prevertebral space involvement
  2. Carotid encased
  3. Mediastinal spread.

  N and M staging as in supraglottis.

When does glottic mass restrict vocal cord mobility?

1. Involvement of thyroarytenoid muscle.
2. Involvement of cricoarytenoid joint.
3. Mass effect.
4. Involvement of recurrent laryngeal nerve (rare).

Investigation as in chapter 16.

What are the radiological findings in paraglottic space involvement?

1. Space between false cords and pyriform fossa is increased.
2. The subglottic contour is reversed in inferior part of paraglottic space involvement.

Paraglottic space is involved in masses which arise from:

i. False cord
ii. Ventricle
iii. True cord
iv. Pyriform fossa (medial wall).

What is carcinoma in situ?

It can occur as:
1. Small limited white patch on cord.
2. Extensive greyish white membrane over larynx.
3. Same as (2) with reddish tinge
   (2) and (3) are more dangerous than T_1 glottis cancer.

Leukoplakia can show:
1. Keratosis (keratinization of superficial layer).
2. Parakeratosis (nuclei retained in keratin layer).
3. Dyskeratosis (keratinization of prickle cell layer).
4. Dysplasia (disorder in epithelial structuring/nuclear mitosis).
5. Carcinoma in situ basement membrane is intact but cells show cytoplasmic/nuclear distortion.

What is lymphatic watershed?

Supraglottis develops from buccopharyngeal anlage III and IV arches and glottis and subglottis from pulmonary analge. So lymphatic drainage is different for the two regions.

Supraglottis drains into level II and III, whereas glottis and subglottis drain into level IV and VI.

Glottis is considered to have very few lymphatics and so there is no nodal involvement in glottic cancers.

What is glottis?

True cord, anterior commissure and posterior commissure.

Lower level of glottis is a horizontal plane one centimeter inferior to the upper surface of the vocal cord. Anatomically true cord extends from superior arcuate line to inferior arcuate line which represents areas on the superior and inferior surface of the cords where squamous epithelium meets respiratory epithelium. Between superior and inferior arcuate line, 5 mm is the vertical height.

How does glottic cancer spread?

1. Via Rienke's space.
2. To anterior commissure and opposite cord.
3. To supraglottis.
4. To subglottis.
5. Once anterior commissure is involved, spread can occur along vertical plane upwards to supraglottis and downwards to subglottis.

Laryngeal cancer spreads to other parts of the larynx by:
a. Direct spread
b. Spreads to mucosa/submucosa and adjacent structures
c. Lymphatics

d. Vascular
e. Perineural.

What prevents spread of glottic cancer?

1. Conus elasticus.
2. Thyroglottic ligament.
3. Vocal ligament.

If cord is mobile, only Reinke's Space is involved.
Investigation as in previous case (chapter 16).

How do you perform direct laryngoscopy?

Direct laryngoscopy is usually performed under general anesthesia. The patient is in a supine position with neck flexed and extension at atlanto axial joint (Boyce's position).

Direct laryngoscopy helps to look at the lesion as well as all hidden areas of the larynx not seen on indirect laryngoscopy.

1. Look for size, site extension of tumor.
2. Look for hidden areas of the larynx such anterior commissure, ventricle, apex of pyriform fossa and subglottic region.
3. Look for vocal cord fixation.
4. Extension to tongue/hypopharynx.
5. Fixation of prevertebral fascia.
6. Pre and paraglottic spaces.
7. Biopsy can be taken. The area should not be one with normal tissue, nor should it be from necrotic material.

If a tracheostomy is needed, it should be done as high as possible at tracheal ring one or two, so that it gets included in Gluck Sorenson's incision.

Complications:

1. Postoperative aspiration as patient is recovering from anesthesia. The best way to prevent this is to have good hemostasis, wait for patient to recover completely before extubating, as cough reflex will be present.
2. Injury to oral cavity and cervical spine.

Contraindications:

1. Rigid endoscopes cannot be used in patients with cervical spine problems.
2. Cannot be done if there are anuerysmal arteries.
3. If patient has trismus, it is difficult to do rigid endoscopy.

What is the treatment for this patient?

Radiotherapy or partial laryngectomy. In this case, vertical extended frontolateral hemilaryngectomy by open method or by endoscopy.
Radiotherapy for $T_2 N_0$ 60 Gy conventional fraction fractionation of 2 Gy.
Surgery:

Endoscopic resection.
Microlaryngeal/cold steel instruments or laser. Endoscope should have a right angled anterior pole to reach anterior commissure. It is possible to do an enbloc anterolateral resection endoscopically.

Describe vertical partial laryngectomy

Collar incision.
Elevate flaps from hyoid to tracheal ring two. Separate sternohyoid and strap muscles only on involved side. Cut muscles off the thyroid cartilage. Incision along superior border of thyroid cartilage to notch and then down midline.

In this case, since tumor involves anterior commissure, entry is not made in the midline. After delineating tumor, cut is made through cricothyroid membrane near the thyroid cartilage and another through the thyrohyoid membrane and the specimen is removed.

Complications:
- Surgical emphysema
- Laryngeal stenosis.

What are other conservative (voice preserving) surgeries?

- Near total laryngectomy
- Supracricoid laryngectomy.

Supracricoid larygectomy:
- Contraindications
  1. Fixed arytenoids.
  2. Subglottic extension.
  3. Posterior commissure involvement.
  4. Tumor involving outer perichondrium of thyroid cartilage.

Resection involves:
- Both vocal cords
- Both false cords
- Both paraglottic spaces
- _+ epiglottis
- Entire thyroid cartilage.

It preserves:
- ? Epiglottis if not removed
- Cricoid cartilage
- One arytenoid
- Hyoid bone.

Release pyriform fossa from thyroid cartilage. Disarticulate cricothyroid joint. Do cricothyrotomy above cricoid cartridge. Incise thyrohyoid membrane. Slit thyroid cartilage. Reposition pyriform fossa.
The larynx is closed by impacting cricoid to hyoid and tongue base thus performing a cricohyoidoepiglottopexy.

No tracheostomy after surgery.

Near total laryngectomy:
One half of the larynx is removed with two-thirds of the other side, leaving one arytenoid and part of vocal cord. A small tube is fashioned with the remaining larynx and arytenoids. Tracheostomy is needed but voice is good. Aspiration is not a frequent occurrence.

Describe total laryngectomy

- Gluck Sorreson's incision
- Identify medial border of sternomastoid muscle
- Identify carotid canal
- Divide strap muscles at the lower limit
- Ligate superior laryngeal bundle. Hypoglossal nerve should be spared
- Clear nodes in level IV and VI
- Hyoid bone held with Allis forceps and cautery used to divide muscle attached to it
- Divide thyroid isthmus and lift the opposite lobe away from the specimen
- Divide the trachea
- Endotracheal tube is transferred to trachea
- It is better to separate larynx from above downwards as interior of larynx is seen
- Holding hyoid bone with a thick forceps, pharynx is opened. The epiglottis is grasped with a forceps and dissection is made along the aryepiglottic folds to reach posterior part of larynx
- The mucosa is divided over the cricoid cartilage
- Divide the inferior constrictor muscle along the sides. The larynx is now separated
- Separate larynx trachea from esophagus
- A small fistula is made between esophagus and tracheostome and a Foley's catheter inserted
- Pharynx is closed with Connell stitches. This picks submucosa but does not pierce mucosa and forms an inverting suture
- Complications:
    1. Pharyngeal fistula occurs between 7-10 days. Wait for 3 weeks; it usually heals.
    2. Narrowing of tracheostome.
    3. Stomal recurrence.

Describe voice rehabilitation after laryngectomy.

The various methods available should be judged on expense to patient, effort by patient, quality of voice.

1. Electronic larynx
   Expense to patient—Moderate
   Effort by patient—No learning curve, can be used in the immediate postoperative period.
   Quality of voice—Poor/electronic.

2. Esophageal speech
   Expense to patient—Has to see speech pathologist.
   Effort by patient—Learning curve variable, not everyone is able to belch air out of esophagus to produce speech.
   Quality of voice—Fairly good, but cannot be sustained for long as air belched from esophagus is nowhere near lung capacity.
3. Tracheoesophageal shunt
   Expense to patient—Primary (if done during first surgery, it is negligible)
   Secondary—A second surgery is needed.
   Removable shunts are less expensive than indwelling shunts.
   Effort by patient—If fistula leaks or gets colonized by fungus, then patient has problems.
   Quality of voice—Good.

What causes poor prognosis in laryngeal cancers?

1. Transglottic/fixed cord.
2. Bilateral nodes/fixed nodes.

What influences distant metastasis?

1. N stage.
2. T stage.
3. Total stage.
4. Histopathology.
5. Presence of recurrent disease after radical treatment.
6. Tumor volume.
7. Alteration of tumor environment by matrix metalloproteases which aids stromal and blood vessel penetration and hence distant metastasis.

What are the symptoms of laryngeal cancer?

1. Progressive hoarseness.
2. Dyspnea and stridor.
3. Dysphagia.
4. Otalgia.
5. Neck swelling.
6. Vague symptoms of food sticking/have to clear throat repeatedly/itchy feeling in the throat.

What will stroboscope show in laryngeal cancer?

1. Inadequate glottic closure.
2. Reduced amplitude of vibration.
3. Distorted mucosal wave.

What are the fallacies in TNM Classification in glottic cancer?

1. Cord fixed is a subjective observation. Everyone need not agree on this.
2. Tumor volume is not taken into consideration.

3. In staging $T_3 N_0$, $T_1 N_2$ are both stage III, but do not have same prognosis.
4. Glottic T_3 includes fixed cord/spread to supraglottis/subglottis.
   Fixed cord has better prognosis and can be treated with CTRT and organ preservation.
   Transglottic tumor has worse prognosis.
5. If anterior commissure is involved, tumor can spread upwards and downwards so calling it anything less than T_3 is not feasible.

How do you treat glottic cancer?

$T_1 T_2 N_0$:
  i. Endoscopic laser resection
  ii. Endoscopic or open partial laryngectomy
  iii. RT

$T_3 N_0$:
i. CTRT
ii. Surgery

Laryngectomy + Hemithyroidectomy ± Neck dissection
T_3N_1 same as $T_3 N_0$ with ipsilateral neck dissection

$T_3 N_{2-3}$: Laryngectomy + Hemithyroidectomy + Bilateral neck dissection or CTRT
$T_4 N_{1-3}$: Total laryngectomy + Hemithyroidectomy + Bilateral neck dissection + CTRT
If patient refuses surgery: CTRT or Induction chemotherapy with CTRT.

What is the behavior of subglottic tumors?

It is rare.

It can be primarily from subgolttis or extension from glottis. It is an ulceroproliferative mass. Invasion of perichondrium and thyroid and cricoid cartilages occur. It can also invade cricothyroid membrane. Cord fixation by spreading to muscles through conus elasticus.

Presenting symptom stridor.

What is the differential diagnosis of squamous cell carcinoma of vocal cord?

1. Tuberculosis.
2. Chronic laryngitis.
3. Benign tumors such as papilloma.
4. Verrucous carcinoma.

Can prognosis of tumor be assessed by histopathology of tumor?

- Basaloid squamous cell carcinoma is more aggressive than squamous cell carcinoma
- Verrucous carcinoma is low grade

- More over tumors can be graded histological (G)
- Gx grade cannot be assessed
- G1 well differentiated
- G2 moderately differentiated
- G3 poorly differentiated
- G4 undifferentiated.

Border's classification of grading tumors histologically:

- 0–25 grade I more differentiated
- 25–50 grade II
- 50–75 grade III
- 75–100 grade IV least differentiated.

The numbers indicate ratio of differentiated and undifferentiated cells.

Can Da Vinci's surgical robot be used in treatment of carcinoma larynx?

- Surgical robot has 3D optics
- It gives a wide view high definition image
- Motor control is good
- Rotational optics is better than line of sight visualization
- It causes enbloc resection, as opposed to piecemeal resection of micro-laryngeal surgery and laser
- Base tongue and supraglottic tumors can be resected endoscopically with robotic 3D.

Chapter 18

Laryngopharyngeal Carcinoma

A 50-year-old man who has a clerical job in a government office presents with pain in the left ear—1 month.
Feeling of foreign body sensation in the throat—3 months.

HISTORY OF PRESENT ILLNESS

Patient says that he has ear pain only in the left ear since 1 month. It is present all the time, mostly dull aching in nature, but sometimes, it is excruciating for a short duration of 2–3 seconds. It started a month ago and has been at the same intensity since then. He has seen a doctor for the same and has been advised ear drops and tablets but there has been no permanent relief. No history of ear discharge, hard of hearing, tinnitus or vertigo. No history of upper respiratory tract infection.
(Ear pain can be associated with Eustachian tube dysfunction)
or
It can be refered pain.
He also has a feeling of a foreign body sensation in the throat for the past 3 months. He says that he keeps swallowing frequently to get rid of the sensation. It was mild previously, but now it is more noticeable. He says that he has no dysphagia, but on enquiry he realises that he has been making his food softer, so that he can swallow more easily.
(In progressive difficulty in swallowing patients overcome the problem by making the food softer and they do not realize it.)

Do you have any acid reflux, heart burn?

No.
(GERD can also cause mild dysphagia and foreign body sensation).

Do you aspirate?/Is there aspiration of undigested food?

No.
(This is seen in pharyngeal pouch).

Is there any weight loss?

May be, I have not weighed myself.

Do you have any difficulty in swallowing liquids?

No.
(In neurological problems, solids can be swallowed as weight of food propels it downwards whereas patients find it more difficult to swallow liquids).

Has there been any trauma to the upper aerodigestive tract?

No.
(Surgery for foreign body removal, history of foreign body which might have caused trauma, history of bouginage for stricture dilatation).

Has there been any cardiovascular incident, central nervous systems disorders?

No.
(These can cause dysphagia).

Is there chest pain?

No.
(30% of chest pain is due to esophageal causes).

Is there a problem in initiating swallowing?

No.
(Pain due to lesions in oral cavity, esophagus, and laryngopharynx may make a patient hesitant to swallow. He resists initiating the effort. In children, it presents as drooling).

- No history of change in voice
- No history of stridor
- No history of any other swelling in the neck.

Past history: No history of past trauma to neck, or surgery of neck. No history of diabetes, hypertension.
Family history: Not significant.
Personal history: Patient is an occasional smoker and drinks everyday. (Quantity is large according to him, may be more than 100 mL/day of country liquor.)
Mixed diet.

From the history what do you think it is?

Maybe an obstructive lesion in the aerodigestive tract with referred otalgia.

Why do you think it is referred otalgia?

There are no other associated ear symptoms; moreover otalgia of a month's duration is not seen in inflammatory ear diseases.

- **General examination**: NAD
- **ENT examination:**

Oral cavity: Normal/no pigmentation of oral cavity mucosa/dental hygiene good.

Dental formula $\frac{2211\ \ 2123}{2211\ \ 0122}$

Oropharynx: No palatal paralysis; gag reflex is present, no other abnormality seen.

Indirect laryngoscopy:- posterior one-third of tongue normal. Valleculla, epiglottis normal. There is an ulcero proliferative mass seen in the left pryiform fossa which is about 2.5 cm in greatest dimension occupying the medial wall; the left arytenoids architecture is maintained even though the growth extends up to the arytenoid. The growth does not extend to posterior part of interarytenoid area, but stops at arytenoid. It does not involve the lateral wall of pyriform fossa, but it is seen occupying the whole of the pyriform fossa.

The arytenoids, the aryepiglottic folds and pharyngoepiglottic folds on both sides are normal.

The right pyriform fossa is normal.

Both false and true cords appear normal.

Pooling of saliva is seen in the left pyriform fossa, but not in the right. *(Chevaliar Jackson's sign)*

On phonation, both cords normal in mobility.

Examination of the neck: Laryngeal architecture is normal. Bocca's sign negative.

Thyroid gland not palpable.

There are 2 swellings palpable on the left side of the neck above the level of hyoid bone between larynx and sternomastoid muscle. The upper swelling is 3 cm in greatest dimension and hard, mobile in all directions.

The lower swelling is 1.5 cm in greatest dimension, hard, mobile in all directions

- The swellings are not warm, tender or pulsatile
- No other palpable swelling in the neck
- Both ears are normal
- Tuning fork test shows no hearing loss
- No facial paralysis
- No signs of vestibular failure
- Nose and sinuses are normal.

Diagnosis: Malignancy of left pyriform fossa with secondaries in the neck (level II) with? referred otalgia.

What is the incidence of various hypopharyngeal malignancies?

- Pyriform fossa—43%
- Postcricoid region—43%
- Posterior pharyngeal wall—9%
- Cervical esophagus—5%.

What is the stage?

- $T_2 N_{2b} M_x$
- Stage IV A.

What is the TNM classification for hypopharynx?

- T_1: Tumor limited to one subsite of hypopharynx/and or 2 cm or less in greatest dimension
- T_2: Tumor invades more than one subsite of hypopharynx or an adjacent site or measures more than 2 cm but less than 4 cm in greatest dimension without fixation of hemilarynx
- T_3: Tumor more than 4 cm in greatest dimension, or with fixation of larynx, or extension to esophagus
- T_{4a}: Moderately advanced local diseases. Tumor invades thyroid/cricoid cartilage/hyoid bone/thyroid gland or central compartment soft tissue (includes prelaryngeal strap muscles and subcutaneous fat)
- T_{4b}: Very advanced local disease. Tumor invades prevertebral fascia. Encases carotid artery or involves mediastinal structures.

Stage I:	$T_1 N_0 M_0$
Stage II:	$T_2 N_0 M_0$
Stage III:	$T_3 N_0 M_0$
	$T_1 N_1 M_0$
	$T_2 N_1 M_0$
	$T_3 N_1 M_0$
Stage IV a:	$T_{4a} N_0 M_0$
	$T_{4a} N_1 M_0$
	$T_1 N_2 M_0$
	$T_2 N_2 M_0$
	$T_3 N_2 M_0$
	$T_{4a} N_2 M_0$
Stage IV b:	T_{4b} Any N M_0
	Any T $N_3 M_0$
Stage IV c:	Any T Any N M_1.

What are the subsites of the hypopharyx?

1. Pyriform sinus: The lateral wall is the thyroid cartilage inner surface and it continuous with the posterior pharyngeal wall. The medial wall is formed by the lateral surface of the arytenoids and merges posteriorly with the postcricoid space. Superior limit is the pharyngoepiglottic fold, and lower limit is the apex situated at the level of the cricoid cartilage.
2. Posterior pharyngeal wall: Extends from the hyoid bone to the cricoid cartilage lower border and from the apex of one pyriform fossa to the other.
3. Postcricoid region: It has only an anterior wall and extends from the posterior surface of the arytenoids to the inferior border of the cricoid cartilage.

How does hypopharyngeal cancer spread?

Pyriform fossa medial wall spreads to aryepiglottic fold to larynx. It can involve the cricoarytenoid joint. It can spread via cricothyroid membrane extralaryngeally. 50% have vocal cord fixation. It has early neck metastasis due to the rich lymphatics in the pyriform fossa. It can spread to cervical esophagus.

Lateral wall tumors can spread to thyroid cartilage, particularly if cartilage in ossified and then to thyroid gland.

Recurrent laryngeal nerve can be involved in apex tumors.

It can also involve base tongue and lateral pharyngeal wall.

Postcricoid tumors can spread to cricoid cartilage, trachea, posterior cricoarytenoid muscle, involve cricothyroid membrane, thyroid gland. It can spread to cervical esophagus submucosally. One third of patients have vocal cord palsy.

Posterior pharyngeal wall spreads to oropharynx, tonsil, it can spread to prevertebral fascia posteriorly.

How does vocal cord palsy occur in pyriform fossa tumors?

1. Cricoarytenoid joint involvement.
2. Posterior cricoarythenoid muscle involvement.
3. Spread to paraglottic space.
4. Recurrent laryngeal nerve involvement.

What is the lymphatic drainage of hypopharynx?

- 70% drain to level II nodes
- 23% to level III and IV
- Pyriform fossa—upper deep cervical: 70–80%
- Postcricoid—upper deep cervical: 30%. It can drain to superior mediastinal nodes
- Posterior pharyngeal wall retropharyngeal nodes and neck nodes
- Upper esophagus—neck nodes and mediastinal nodes.

Where does it metastatize?

- Lung
- Liver
- Bones
- Oropharyngeal tumors can have a second primary in the pyriform fossa
- Pyriform fossa tumors can have a second primary in the lungs.

What are the symptoms of hypopharyngeal tumor?

- Dysphagia: Early in postcriocoid/late in pyriform fossa
- Hoarseness of voice
- Sore throat
- Otalgia through vagus nerve
- Neck nodes
- Pain on swallowing

- Unilateral sore throat
- Globus.

What are the predisposing causes of hypopharyngeal tumors?

- Smoking
- Alcohol
- Low intake of fresh fruits and vegetables
- Low zinc in the diet
- Low vitamin C and vitamin E
- Welding fumes
- Exposure to irradiation
- Plummer-Winson's syndrome.

What is Plummer-Winson's syndrome?

This is usually a woman patient who has angular stomatitis, koilonychia, iron deficiency and web in the postcricoid region or web between postcricoid region and thoracic esophagus. Web is initially anterior and later becomes circumferential.

Initially dysphagia is intermittent, and later constant. Patient modifies diet to softer food.

If it is not managed by iron and vitamins, 30% have a risk of developing postcricoid malignancies.

How will you investigate this patient with pyriform fossa mass?

1. X-ray neck lateral view
2. CT/MRI of neck. In hypopharynx MRI may be superior, but it shows peritumor edema and so tumor size is over estimated. CT may underestimate size.
3. CT of the chest: Since there is a great chance of a second primary in the lung, a CT of the chest is better than an X-ray chest because CT shows second primaries which are 3 mm in size whereas chest X-ray shows tumors which are 1–2 cm in size.

How will you know if it is a second primary or a secondary in the chest?

- Large neck nodes are likely to cause a secondary
- In the presence of small neck nodes, one has to assume it is a second primary in the chest.

Does the final outcome depend on whether it is a second primary or secondary in the lung?

If lung disease is operable it makes no difference.

4. Pan endoscopy:
   a. Full inspection of oral cavity and oropharynx with a tonsil gag

b. Palpate posterior one-third of tongue.
c. Examine postnasal space with zero degree endoscope.
d. Use Lindholm endoscope to get a wide view of lower oropharynx and laryngopharynx.
e. Laryngeal ventricles should be examined with an angled Hopkin's rod telescope.
f. Complete laryngoscopy. It is important to look for cord mobility and to check size and extent of tumor. Upper limit of tumor has to be assessed and biopsy taken.
g. Check for prevertebral fascia involvement by moving the end of the scope on the prevertebral fascia.
h. Esophagoscopy with a fiberoptic instrument can be done. If mass is seen, a rigid scopy and biopsy should follow.
i. Bronchoscopy.

5. Dental checkup.
6. Nutrition and speech pathologist.

How will you treat this patient?

- Organ preservation treatment is possible.
- Larynx is not involved.
- So, either CTRT or induction chemotherapy with CTRT can be tried.
- If CTRT is given cisplatin 100 mg/mm^2 x 3 doses every 3 weeks + RT
- 66–74 Gy to primary and involved neck
- 44–64 Gy to uninvolved neck.

If after CTRT primary site shows residual tumor, then partial laryngopharyngectomy can be done.
If after CTRT primary is cleared but neck nodes persist, neck dissection can be done.

How will you treat hypopharyngeal malignancies?

T_2N_0 }
T_2N_0 } Radiotherapy or partial laryngopharygectomy + neck dissection

T_1N^+ }
T_2N^+, T_3N^+ and }
$T_{4a}N^+$ } surgery laryngopharyngectomy + neck dissection or CTRT

T_3T_4 tumors need postoperative irradiation after 3–6 weeks.
Irradiation dose:

- Primary site: 60–66 Gy
- Involved neck: 60–66 Gy
- Uninvolved neck: 44–66 Gy.

What are the complications of radiotherapy?

a. Mucositis
b. Skin damage

c. Reduced salivary flow
d. Radiation induced laryngeal edema
e. Chondronecrosis
f. Postcricoid irradiation can lead to strictures.

What is Partial Pharyngectomy?

I. Partial pharyngectomy can be done as the only procedure for very small (T_1) tumors of posterior pharyngeal wall or medial wall of pyriform fossa.
   1. Lateral pharyngotomy: Thyroid ala is exposed laterally and posteriorly, inferior constrictor muscle is cut and pharynx entered. Mass is excised and primary closure is possible.
   2. Lateral transhyoid pharyngotomy:
      - Here pharynx is entered through vallecula. Posterior part of thyroid ala and part of hyoid is removed to get adequate margin.
   3. Anterior transhyoid pharyngotomy: Done in T_1 T_2 posterior pharyngeal wall tumors.
      Collar incision is made in the neck, hyoid identified and resected, and vallecula entered. Inferior traction of pharynx and superior traction of base tongue exposes posterior pharyngeal wall mass. Tumor excised and wound closed with skin graft.
   4. Median labiomandibular glossotomy:
      - Lip splitting incision down to mandible and inferiorly upto hyoid.
      - Tongue is split in an avascular plane to reach posterior pharyngeal wall.

II. Partial pharyngectomy and near total laryngectomy can be done for more extensive tumors which have spread to marginal zone, supraglottis and if cord is fixed. Closure is possible without graft.
   Resected specimen has
   a. Medial wall of pyriform fossa
   b. Ipsilateral arytenoids
   c. Ipsilateral half of hyoid
   d. Superior 2/3 of ipsilateral thyroid cartilage.

   Reconstruction can be done with regional flap (pectoralis major myocutaneous flap or radial forearm free flap).
   Contraindications:
   1. Pyriform fossa apex involvement
   2. Postcricoid involvement.

III. Total laryngectomy with total pharyngectomy
   Here pharynx can be replaced with a jejunal flap/radial forearm flap. Success is best with jejunal flap even though it requires abdominal surgery.
   Total laryngectomy with total pharyngectomy is indicated in the following cases.
   1. Pyriform fossa tumors extending to postcricoid region.
   2. If posterior pharyngeal wall mass extends to pyriform fossa.
   3. Most postcricoid tumors.

IV. Total laryngectomy with pharyngectomy with esophagectomy
Best replacement is stomach (gastric pull up).
Indicated in larger postcricoid and cervical esophagus lesions.
Gastric pull up leads to death because of
1. Pneumonia/pneumothorax (insertion of chest drains can prevent this).
2. Graft necrosis.
3. Anastomotic leak.
4. Hemorrhage *(A diverticuloscope can be used in the middle mediastinum to prevent this)*
5. Myocardial infarction.
6. Cardiovascular accident.
7. Respiratory failure.
8. Tracheal necrosis.

V. Supracricoid hemilaryngectomy: This can be done for medial wall of pyriform fossa or hypopharyngeal aspect of aryepiglottic fold if patient has good pulmonary reserve and apex of pyriform fossa is not involved.

What are the causes of failure in hypopharyngeal cancer?

- No difference between radiation and surgery.
- Postcricoid and pyriform fossa | 46% success
- Postpharyngeal wall is worse
- Cervical esophagus bad.

Here T_1 is better than T_4 but T_2 and T_3 there is no difference.

Number of nodes and extracapsular spread is important. Contralateral nodes and extracapsular spread have bad prognosis.

- Tumor less than 4 cm has 50% lymph node spread
- Tumor more than 4 cm has 85% nodal metastasis.

Surgical margin should be 2 cm because of submucosal infiltration upto 1 cm.

Chapter 19

Thyroid Neoplasm

A 45-year-old man presents with a swelling in front of the neck—3 months, Hoarseness of voice—1 month.

HISTORY OF PRESENT ILLNESS

Patient says that the swelling was the size of a lemon to start with and over the past month it has increased in size rapidly.
(Patient explains in his terminology, e.g. size of a lemon, cricket ball, pea, etc.)
Rapid increase in size can be due to hemorrhage into the swelling.
Rapid increase in size also suggests malignant change.

The swelling started on the right side of the neck and is also seen in front now.
(Swellings in the anterior part of the neck can be lateral or in the midline.)

Lateral swellings	*Midline swellings*
Branchial cyst	Thyroglossal cyst
Lymph nodes	Lymph nodes
Lateral lobe of thyroid	Swelling in the isthmus of thyroid gland
Parapharyngeal tumors	Subhyoid bursitis
External laryngocele	
Pharyngeal pouch	

Is it or has it ever been associated with pain?

No.

Painful swellings	*Painless swellings*
Acute/subacute thyroidtis	Goiter
Infected branchial cyst	Tuberculous lymph nodes
Suppurative lymph nodes	Secondary neck nodes
Perichondritis of thyroid cartilage	Noninfected branchial cyst
Hemorrhage into a thyroid nodule	Laryngocele
	Pharyngeal pouch

Have you had accidental or operation trauma in the head and neck region?

No.
Neck abscesses can present as swelling in the neck and it can follow tonsillectomy, dental extraction, etc.

Is there fever, evening rise of temperature, night sweats, loss of weight or appetite?

No.

- *Tuberculous lymphadenitis can cause any of the above symptoms*
- *Loss of weight in spite of a good appetite is seen in thyrotoxicosis*
- *Pharyngeal pouch can also result in loss of weight*
- *Significant loss of weight is losing 10% of the weight in 6 months.*

Does the swelling increase in size during deglutition?

No.
Pharyngeal pouches increase in size during deglutition.

Is there a change in size during inspiration?

No.
External laryngoceles vary in size during respiration.

Has your hoarseness progressed?

Yes, my voice was perfectly normal a month ago, but now it has gradually become weak.

Gradual pressure on the recurrent laryngeal nerve initially causes cough and regurgitation. Later, it results in a whispered voice. Compensation occurs later (Refer to the case presentation on hoarseness of voice for other details).

Do you have difficulty in swallowing?

No.
Pressure over the esophagus can cause dysphagia.

Do you have difficulty in breathing?

No.
Pressure over trachea can cause stridor.

Do you have increased (voracious) appetite, loss of weight, palpation, diarrhea, intolerance to heat?

No.
These are symptoms of hyperthyroidism; diarrhea can also occur in medullary carcinoma due to increased calcitonin and ACTH like substances.

Have you put on weight, do you feel weak, have hair loss, constipation, anorexia, vomiting, intolerance to cold?

No.
These are symptoms of hypothyroidism.

Do you have hearing loss; dizziness, tinnitus?

No.
These occur because of accumulation of glycosaminoglycans in the cochlea, vestibule. Also in the vocal cords, this produces voice change (seen in hypothyroidism)

PAST HISTORY

Is there any history of diabetes, hypertension, asthma, allergies, epilepsy?

No.

Did you have any previous surgeries in the neck?

No.
- *Present swelling may be a neoplastic change in a previously operated nodular goiter*
- *Patient might have undergone surgeries for laryngeal malignancies.*

Have you ever been irradiated with ^{131}I or any form of irradiation, accidental leak of nuclear material?

No.
- *Can be an etiological factor in thyroid malignancies*
- *Accidental irradiation as in Chernobyl disaster increased thyroid carcinoma particularly in children.*

Have you been on prolonged medication for any diseases?

No.
Drugs like amiodarone, lithium and antithyroid drugs can cause goiter.

Do you have diabetes or hypertension?

No.
Diastolic hypertension is seen in hypothyroidism and systolic hypertension is seen in hyperthyroidism.

FAMILY HISTORY

Are there any other family members who have neck swelling or have been treated in the past for the same?

No.
- *Genetic factors are important as even in endemic area for goiter, some families have it while others don't*
- *Some medullary carcinomas are familial.*

PERSONAL HISTORY

Do you consume millets cassava, cabbage frequently?

Yes.
These can prevent uptake of iodine.

Do you smoke?

Yes.
Smoking is known to prevent uptake of iodine.

DISCUSSION

What is your diagnosis after history taking?

It may be a neoplasm of the thyroid gland probably malignant.
Reasons

- Short duration
- Patient points to the anatomical region of the thyroid gland
- Swelling appeared to be too small to cause pressure over recurrent laryngeal nerve by mechanical means. So, it may have infiltrated the nerve to cause hoarseness.

Can it be a lymph node?

It cannot be ruled out. There is history of hoarseness indicating involvement of the larynx.

Can it be tuberculosis?

There is no history suggestive of tuberculosis.

General examination

Refer earlier cases.

Examination of the neck

(For details of neck examination, see chapter 24).

Inspection

There is a swelling in the region of the right lobe of thyroid extending from the hyoid bone to the suprasternal notch. It extends horizontally from the anterior border of the right sternomastoid muscle to the midline along the lower border of the cricoid and first tracheal ring on to the left lobe of the thyroid gland. It does not extend to the anterior border of the left sternomastoid muscle.

- *A normal thyroid gland is not visible on inspection. A thyroid gland is enlarged if it is larger than the terminal phalanx of the thumb of the person being examined*

The lower border of the swelling is seen
- *If the lower border of the swelling is not seen even on extension of the head a retrosternal extension is possible. In such cases if patient raises his arm above his head and maintains the position for some time, then there may be facial suffusion or respiratory distress (Pemberton's sign)*
- *If the patient has short neck than Pizzillo's method can be used to examine the thyroid gland. Clasped hands of the patient is placed behind his occiput and patient is asked to push neck and against his clasped hands*

The skin over the swelling is normal

The swelling moves with deglutition
- *This is because the pretracheal fascia splits to enclose the thyroid gland, so when the trachea moves thyroid gland also moves*

The swelling does not move on protrusion of the tongue
- *Thyroglossal cyst moves on protrusion of the tongue Thyroglossal cyst moves on protrusion of the tongue because the thyroglossal duct extends downwards from the foramen cecum to the isthmus of the thyroid gland*

There are no other swellings or sinuses in the neck on inspection
- *Neck nodes may be enlarged in papillary, medullary and anaplastic thyroid malignancies*

The laryngeal architecture appears normal, there is no tracheal shift
- *Large thyroid swellings can displace trachea.*

Palpation

- On palpation, the swelling measures 5 x 4 cm
- It is hard and all the margins are palpable
- Skin over the swellings is free
- The swelling does not involve the sternomastoid muscle
- It involves the right lobe of thyroid, the isthmus and a centimeter of the left lobe
- The lateral margin of the left lobe is not enlarged
- The surface is smooth; there are no sinuses over the swelling
- It is not warm, tender or compressible
- No dilated veins over the swelling
- On applying pressure over the left tracheal groove, the lateral margin of the right lobe can be palpated
- No enlargement of the pyramidal lobe.

There is a second swelling just lateral to the right thyroid lobe. It is situated between the hyoid and cricoid cartilages at the position of level 3 node. The swelling is 2 x 1 cm, hard in consistency, not tender not compressible and freely mobile.

There are no other swellings or sinuses in the neck.

The trachea is in the midline and the laryngeal frame work is normal; the carotid pulsations are felt.

Placing a thumb on the thyroid gland on the right side, the patient was asked to swallow. No nodules are palpable *(This is Crile's method to palpate nodules that are not easily palpable).*

- *Palpation of thyroid reveals the following characteristics*
  Multinodular goiter—smooth nodularity
  Malignant—firm nodules
  Colloid nodules—doughy
  Autoimmune disease—fine bosselated appearance
  Papillary and medullary carcinomas—hard and rubbery
  Carcinoma—hard fixed craggy
  Lymphoma—smooth diffuse
  Cystic swelling may feel firm when tense; and hard when calcified.

Examination of the oral cavity/oropharynx

- No lingual thyroid swelling
- *Fibrillations of tongue are seen in thyrotoxicosis*
- *Thick tongue is seen in hypothyroidism.*

Indirect laryngoscopy

The right vocal cord is paralyzed and is in the paramedian position. There is no pooling of saliva or edema of the arytenoids. No other mass seen.

Examination of the eye specific to thyroid

No evidence of Horner's syndrome or any other eye signs
Horner's syndrome

- *Sinking of the eyeball—enopthalmos*
- *Sight drooping of upper eyelid—ptosis*
- *Contraction of pupils—miosis*
- *Absence of sweat on the affected side—anhidrosis.*

Some classical eye signs in thyrotoxicosis

- Eyelid retraction—upper lid is higher than normal, lower lid is normal. (This is due to over activity of involuntary part of levator palpabrae superiors muscle)
- Lid lag—upper eyelid cannot keep pace with the eyeball where patient looks down (von Graefe's sign)
- Exophthalmoses—eyeball is pushed forwards due to fat, edema and cellular infiltration of retro-orbital fat. Hence, eyelids are retracted and sclera is seen. Upper sclera is visible (Dalrymple's sign)
- Stellwag's sign—Staring look, infrequent blinking, and wide palpebral fissure due to toxic contraction of striated fibers of levator palpebrae superioris
- Ophthalmoplegia—weakness of ophthalmic muscles due to edema and cellular infiltration. Muscles most affected are superior and lateral rectus and inferior oblique
- Chemosis—conjunctival edema.

Cardiovascular system

Clinically normal.

- Tachycardia, increased pulse rate especially increased sleeping pulse rate is confirmatory, irregular pulse, increased blood pressure is seen in hyperthyroidism.

CNS

Clinically normal.

- *Fine tremors and anxiety may be seen in thyrotoxicosis*
- *Delayed ankle reflex may be seen in hypothyroidism.*

Eye signs are mostly seen in primary thyrotoxicosis where as cardiovascular signs are common in secondary thyrotoxicosis.

Examination of the ear

Clinically normal.
(To look for sensorineural hearing loss, vestibular failure, and otitis media with effusion).

Skin

Clinically normal.

- *Moist in hyperthyroidism dry and thick in hyperthyroidism.*

Clinical diagnosis: Malignant lesson of the right thyroid lobe extending to the isthmus and left lobe with secondary cervical node with right vocal cord palsy. Patient is clinically euthyroid.

Why do you think it is thyroid?

Anatomical position and it moves with deglutition.

Why do you think it is malignant?

1. Short duration.
2. Presence of a node.
3. Involvement of vocal cord.
4. Swelling is hard in consistency.

What is the stage?

$T_{4a}N_{1b}Mx$; stage IV A.
Staging varies with the histopathological nature of the malignancy.
Types are:

Differentiated	*Undifferentiated*
Papillary—80%	Anaplastic—2%
Follicular—8%	
Hurtle cell—11%	
Medullary—24%	

TNM staging for thyroid cancer (UICC 2007)

Primary tumor (T)

[Note: All categories may be subdivided into (a) solitary tumor or (b) multifocal tumor (the largest determines the classification).]

- TX: Primary tumor cannot be assessed
- T_0: No evidence of primary tumor
- T_1: Tumor 2 cm or less in greatest dimension, limited to the thyroid
- T_2: Tumor more than 2 cm but not more than 4 cm in greatest dimension, limited to the thyroid
- T_3: Tumor more than 4 cm in greatest dimension limited to the thyroid or any tumor with minimal extrathyroid extension (e.g., extension to sternothyroid muscle or perithyroid soft tissues)
- T_{4a}: Tumor of any size extending beyond the thyroid capsule to invade subcutaneous soft tissues, larynx, trachea, esophagus, or recurrent laryngeal nerve
- T_{4b}: Tumor invades prevertebral fascia or encases carotid artery or mediastinal vessels.

All anaplastic carcinomas are considered T_4 tumors.

- T_{4a}: Intrathyroidal anaplastic carcinoma—surgically resectable
- T_{4b}: Extrathyroidal anaplastic carcinoma—surgically unresectable.

As you can see if the current tumor being examined is anaplastic on histopathological examination it becomes T_{4b} instead of T_{4a}.

Regional lymph nodes (N)

Regional lymph nodes are the central compartment, lateral cervical, and upper mediastinal lymph nodes.

- NX: Regional lymph nodes cannot be assessed
- N_0: No regional lymph node metastasis
- N_1: Regional lymph node metastasis
- N_{1a}: Metastasis to level VI (pretracheal, paratracheal, and prelaryngeal/Delphian lymph nodes)
- N_{1b}: Metastasis to unilateral or bilateral cervical or superior mediastinal lymph nodes.

Distant metastases (M)

MX: Distant metastasis cannot be assessed
M_0: No distant metastasis
M_1: Distant metastasis.

UICC stage groupings

Separate stage groupings are recommended for papillary or follicular, medullary, and anaplastic (undifferentiated) carcinoma.

Papillary or follicular thyroid cancer

Younger than 45 years

- Stage I Any T, any N, M_0
- Stage II Any T, any N, M_1.

Age 45 years and older

- Stage I T_1, N_0, M_0
- Stage II T_2, N_0, M_0
- Stage III T_3, N_0, M_0, T_1, N_{1a}, M_0 , T_2, N_{1a}, M_0, T_3, N_{1a}, M_0
- Stage IVA T_{4a}, N_0, M_0, T_{4a}, N_{1a}, M_0, T_1, N_{1b}, M_0, T_2, N_{1b}, M_0, T_3, N_{1b}, M_0, T_{4a}, N_{1b}, M_0
- Stage IVB T_{4b}, any N, M_0
- Stage IVC Any T, any N, M_1.

Medullary thyroid cancer

- Stage I T_1, N_0, M_0
- Stage II T_2, N_0, M_0
- Stage III T_3, N_0, M_0, T_1, N_{1a}, M_0, T_2, N_{1a}, M_0, T_3, N_{1a}, M_0
- Stage IVA T_{4a}, N_0, M_0, T_{4a}, N_{1a}, M_0, T_1, N_{1b}, M_0, T_2, N_{1b}, M_0, T_3, N_{1b}, M_0, T_{4a}, N_{1b}, M_0
- Stage IVB T_{4b}, any N, M_0
- Stage IVC Any T, any N, M_1.

Anaplastic thyroid cancer

All anaplastic carcinomas are considered stage IV.

- Stage IVA-T_{4a}, any N, M_0
- Stage IVB T_{4b}, any N, M_0
- Stage IVC Any T, any N, M_1.

Thyroid is one site of the head and neck where age and histopathology of tumor is considered in staging along with the size which in the only criteria in other sites.

How will you manage this patient?

(For evaluation of a thyroid nodule please refer case on multinodular goiter)

1. T_3, T_4 and TSH to evaluate thyroid function
   Increased TSH increases risk of differentiated cancer
   TSH is the most sensitive index
   Normal TSH: normal functioning thyroid
   Low TSH with normal T_4 = subclinical hyperthyroidism
   Raised TSH with normal T_4 = subclinical hypothyroidism.
2. Serum thyroglobulin: Increased levels are seen in thyroid cancer, auto immune thyroiditis and viral thyroiditis. It is not raised in medullary cancer.
3. Antithyroid antibodies should be evaluated because antithyroid antibodies lower serum thyroglobulin value falsely. Antithyroid antibodies are raised in autoimmune diseases.
4. Serum calcitonin is raised in medullary carcinoma. False positive test can be ruled out by doing pentagastrin studies.
5. Serum calcium: hypercalcaemia as a part of hyper parathyroidism is seen in multiple endocrine neoplasia 2a (MEN 2a) and MEN 2b medullary carcinoma.
6. RET proto-oncogene mutation in exon 10, 11, 13–16 is seen in papillary and medullary carcinoma. RAS gene activation causing cell proliferation. This is seen in follicular and anaplastic cancer.

BRAF is mutated in papillary carcinoma.
7. CEA is increased in medullary carcinoma.

RADIOLOGY

It is better to do the radiological investigations prior to fine needle aspiration cytology (FNAC) to avoid artifacts.

X-ray chest and neck to look for

1. Tracheal shift
2. Mediastinal extension of thyroid gland
3. Mediastinal lymph nodes
4. Compression of trachea—Scabbard sign
5. Fine calcification of thyroid gland
6. Psammoma bodies—papillary carcinoma
7. Rim of egg shell calcification benign lesson
8. Upper lateral pole calcification sometimes bilateral—medullary carcinoma
9. Irregular calcification multinodular goiter.

Ultrasound of neck

1. To detect nodularity/differentiate between solid and cystic nodules
2. To assess tumor size
3. To assess neck nodes
4. Characteristics on ultrasound which show malignancy of neck nodes are: increase in size with rounded and bulging shape and loss of fatty hilum.

Computed tomography (CT) scan

1. To assess size.
2. Involvement of surrounding structure.
3. Nodes in the neck and mediastinum.
4. Retrosternal extensions.
5. Abdominal CT—pheochromocytoma.
6. Distant metastasis, CNS, bone pulmonary.

MRI Scan

1. Extracapsular extension.
2. Spread to surrounding structures.

Scintigraphy (Thyroid Scan)

^{99m}Tc can be used instead of ^{123}I. ^{99m}Tc is cheaper as it is not cyclotron generated; Radiation is low, trapped by thyroid gland but not organified. ^{123}I is cyclotron generated, taken up by thyroid gland but organified. The advantage is that it is physiologically closer than ^{99m}Tc.

Scintigraph is essential to distinguish

1. Cold or hot (solitary nodule)
2. Ectopic thyroid
3. Suspected malignancies.

^{123}I M1BG scanning (Metaiodobenzylguanidine) is taken up by neural crest derivatives, hence good in medullary carcinoma and gallium scanning is helpful in lymphoma.

FNAC

Histological specimens are classified as:
- Thy 1—inadequate for diagnosis
- Thy 2—benign diseases
- Thy 3—suspicion of neoplasm
- Thy 4—suspicion for malignancy
- Thy 5—positive for malignancy.

Follicular adenoma and follicular carcinoma cannot be differentiated because the differentiating factors such as capsular invasion and vessel invasion cannot be made out in FNAC.

After the investigation and FNAC what do you expect?

Investigation will probably reveal a malignant lesson.

If it is malignant what is your next line of action?

Depending on whether it differentiated or not and based on the histology, I will take the following action:
Patient is male above 45 years, so I will do a total thyroidectomy with clearance of level VI nodes and a modified neck dissection on the right side (II, III, IV) . (Details of surgical procedure of total thyroidectomy can be found in multinodular goiter case chapter)

Treatment plan for papillary carcinoma

Less than 1 cm—lobectomy and isthmusectomy followed by throid-stimulating hormone (TSH) suppression with T_4 replacement.

Anything larger requires total thyroidectomy with level VI resection because (exception can be in women less than 40 who have tumors of 2 cm less-lobectomy)
1. Disease can be multicentric.
2. Recurrent disease is seen after 25 years and it can be more virulent and may be anaplastic carcinoma.
3. Injuring both recurrent laryngeal nerves during surgery should not be a deterrent to doing total thyroidectomy.
4. Doing lobectomy and isthmusectomy and using ^{131}I to destroy the remaining thyroid tissue requires high doses of ^{131}I.
5. Total thyroidectomy can be followed by ^{131}I total body scan to look for local recurrence, node recurrence and distant metastasis.
6. Serum thyroglobulin levels should be estimated regularly after surgery to look for recurrences. This can be effectively done after total thyroidectomy.

Comparison of lobectomy vs total thyroidectomy

After 20 years	*Local recurrence*	*Nodal metastasis*
Lobectomy	14%	19%
Total thyroidectomy	02%	06%

Treatment of cervical nodes

No clinical and radiological nodes—level VI resection. This is essential because nodes from thyroid drain to tracheoesophageal groove, mediastinal nodes, prelaryngeal nodes, and then to the jugular chain. Some lymphatics also pass through the tracheal wall.

Clinically or radiologically positive nodes—lateral neck dissection (II, III, IV) with central compartment clearance.

Treatment plan for follicular tumors

More than 1 cm—total thyroidectomy with level VI clearance

Node enlarged clinically—total thyroidectomy with level VI clearance with modified neck dissection with radioactive 1^{131} ablation of thyroid bed and neck.

Treatment plan for medullary carcinoma

Medullary less than 1 cm—total thyroidectomy with level VI clearance (dissection of nodes from hyoid to innominate vessels and laterally from carotid to carotid).

More than 1 cm—total thyroidectomy with level VI clearance with radical neck dissection with superior mediastinal node clearance to look for recurrence.

Radiotherapy is given in cases of positive margins and in case of gross extrathyroidal disease. Chemotherapy has no role.

What are the types of medullary carcinoma thyroid? When do you investigate for them?

MCT may be classified as follows:

1. Sporadic
2. Familial
   - Familial MCT
   - MEN 2A
   - MEN 2B

Sporadic	*Familial*
80%	20%
Older age—5–6 decades	Younger age—2–3 decades
Unilateral	May be bilateral
Unifocal	Multifocal

No family history	Family history
More in females	Both sex equally affected
May be associated with other parathyroid neoplastic syndromes like diarrhea (prostaglandins and VIP), Cushing syndrome (ACTH)	There are associated tumors I MEN 2A and 2B

Indications to investigate for familial MCT:
- Young age
- Bilateral/multicentric disease
- Clinical features of familial MCT
- Family history of MCT or other tumors associated with MEN.

Investigations for suspected familial MCT:
- Serum calcitonin
- Serum calcium, serum phosphate and serum parathyroid hormone (PTH) for parathyroid tumors
- USG abdomen, urinary vanillylmandelic acid
- CT neck and thorax.

Metastatic work-up for all MCTs:
- Chest X-ray
- USG abdomen
- Bone scan.

Describe the genetics of hereditary MCT

As mentioned above the hereditary form of MCT can present in 3 ways. These case have mutations in RET oncogene on chromosome 10. They have autosomal dominant inheritance.

1. MEN 2A—mutations on codon 634.
2. MEN 2B—mutations on codons 883 and 918. More aggressive of all three.
3. Familial—most indolent of all three.

Depending on the mutations on the RET proto oncogene, prophylactic surgery is undertaken. Mutations on codons 609 and 768—prophylactic thyroidectomy at 5–10 years; 634 and 618—before 5 years and 883 and 918—surgery by 1 year.

How do you look for recurrence in MCT?

Basal calcitonin levels and carcinoembryonic antigen (these are circulating secretory products of medullary carcinoma) should be estimated every 6 to 12 months.

If increased, do contrast enhanced CT or MRI of neck, chest and abdomen with liver protocol.

In the presence of locoregional disease, RT or if possible surgical resection is done.

In case of metastasis, consider RT for local symptoms or small molecule tyrosine kinase inhibitors or dacarbazine based chemotherapy.

Bone metastasis can be treated for palliation with biphosphonates.
CEA is only prognostic and not diagnostic.

What is the treatment for anaplastic carcinoma?

In rare cases, when they are operable, they are treated with total thyroidectomy. In most of the other cases they are given palliative radiotherapy and adriamycin based chemotherapy.

What will you do for distant metastasis (other than MCT)?

Metastasis	*Percentage*	*Treatment options*
Bone	15%	surgical resection, biphosphonate therapy, embolization of bone metastasis
Pulmonary	45%	^{131}I ablation
CNS	10%	Neurosurgical resection, radioactive iodine, image guided radiotherapy

Can thyroid be a site for distant metastasis?

Yes.

- Metastatic renal carcinoma—follicular carcinoma
- Melanoma—medullary carcinoma
- Pulmonary—anaplastic carcinoma of thyroid.

When is ^{131}I Scan done after thyroidectomy?

It can be performed after 4–6 weeks.

What do you expect from ^{131}I Scan?

This is to look for residual tumor in the thyroid bed, residual disease in the neck or distant metastasis.

How do you prepare the patient for ^{131}I Scan?

TSH stimulation (more than 30 mIU) should be adequate, i.e. if patient is on T_4, it should be stopped for at least 4 weeks for TSH level to rise. In addition, all iodine containing drugs like cough expectorants and food stuff like sea food and iodized salt should be withdrawn.

Do all thyroid malignancies take up ^{131}I?

Medullary carcinoma arises from parafollicular cells and hence does not take up I^{131}.

How do you follow up the patient with ^{131}I imaging and ablation after total thyroidectomy?

- Total thyroidectomy is done
- After surgery wait for 4 weeks for TSH level to rise

- Then do a whole body ^{131}I scan
- If residual thyroid tissue is made out on the scan this tissue will have to be abalated by I^{131}
- Repeat scan after 6 months
- Treat with I^{131} till scans are negative and thyroglobulin level is less than 2 ng/mL
- Suppressive treatment with thyroxin and follow up with thyroglobulin and TSH.

How do you treat a positive scan?

Residual neck disease is treated with a dose of 3.7 GBq of ^{131}I.

A range between 1.1 to 3.7 GBq is used but higher dose such as 3.7 GBq gives better results.

After initiating the treatment patient is admitted in an isolation ward for 3 to 6 days.

What are the long-term effects of radioiodine therapy?

In persons who have received high doses, there is a risk of developing leukemia.

What are the contraindications for radioiodine therapy?

- Pregnancy—delay conception for 1 year
- Breastfeeding.

What does prognosis of thyroid cancer depend on?

- Age—less than 45 years
- Sex—women have a better prognosis then men
- Grade of tumor—histologically well differentiated less aggressive tumors
- Extrathyroid invasion—has a worse prognosis
- Distant metastasis—has a worse prognosis
- Size—smaller the size better the prognosis.

Using these factors various institutes have developed criteria to predict prognosis.

- GAMES (Memorial Sloan Kettering)—grade, age, metastasis, extrathyroid extension, size.
- AGES (Mayo clinic)—age, grade, extension, size
- AMES (Lahey clinic)—age, metastasis, extension, size
- DAMES (Karolinska institute)—DNA, age, metastasis, extension, size
- MACIS (Mayo)—metastasis, age, completeness of surgery, extrathyroid invasion, size.

Some of the factors like age and sex are patient factors over which we have no control. Some factors depend on the tumor like size, histology, node or distant metastasis over which again we have no control. The factors over which we have control are the extent and timing of treatment, experience of the surgeon, T_4 replacement and ^{131}I ablation.

Chapter 20

Goiter

A 30-year-old woman presents with a swelling in front of the neck—6 years duration.

HISTORY OF PRESENT ILLNESS

- Swelling was small to start with; it was size of a lemon on the right side of the neck and gradually progressed to the present level
- She has no dysphagia, stridor or hoarseness of voice
- She has no symptoms of hypo or hyperthyroidism. (See history taking in the chapter 19)
- All the questions to be asked as in chapter 19
- She has no other positive history.

LOCAL EXAMINATION

There is a swelling in the anterior aspect of the right side of the neck about 6 x 5 cm. The swelling is in the right tracheoesophageal groove and extends from the hyoid bone to the suprasternal notch. It extends over the airway at the level of the cricoid cartilage and first tracheal ring to the left tracheoesophageal groove. The swelling on the left side is about 4 x 3 cm. On both sides the swelling extends to the sternomastoid muscle anterior border.

Swelling moves with deglutition, it appears smooth and there are no dilated vessels over the swelling.

PALPATION

It measures 6 x 5 cm on the right side and 4 x 3 cm on the left side. Over the air way, it is 1 x 3/4 cm The surface is smooth and interspersed with nodular lesion all over the swelling. Consistency is soft and it is not reducible. No pulsations felt. Trachea is shifted to the left.

- Rest of neck is normal
- No palpable lymph nodes in the neck
- Do the rest of the examination as in the chapter 19.

Diagnosis multinodular goiter involving both lobes of thyroid and the patient is clinically euthyroid.

Can it be malignant?

There is no involvement of neighboring structures like recurrent laryngeal nerve, esophagus and trachea. No history of rapid increase in size.

So why has the patient come to the hospital?

She feels the swelling is large and cosmetically unacceptable to her.

Do you advise surgery?

Yes.
Thyroid swelling can be removed for cosmoses but some investigations have to be done first.

What will you do?

Repeat all investigations as in chapter 19.

Among these, which do you feel is in important here?

1. Ultrasound scanning reveals the nature of nodularity whether it is solid or cystic.
   Solid nodes are more likely to be malignant.
   Microfollicular nodes are hypoechoic whereas macrofollicular nodes are hyperechoic.
   Homogenous hyperechoic lesions with thin hypoechoic rims, and having egg shell calcification are likely to be benign.
   Malignancy is indicated by non-homogeneous echo pattern, solid areas in cystic lesions, central vascularization.
2. Technetium scanning using Tc^{99} will reveal a hot or cold nodule. Hot nodules are benign, cold nodules require rescanning or fine needle aspiration cytology (FNAC). If nodule is solid and cold than chances of malignancy increases.
3. FNAC—results can be difficult to interpret if T_3 T_4 levels are high or low.
   FNAC has 72–100% specificity to detect cancer and 65–98% sensitivity.
   It cannot detect follicular adenoma from carcinoma as this can only be made out by extracapsular invasion and or vessel infiltration.

Can T_3 T_4 TSH help towards diagnosis?

A raised TSH level is suspicious for malignancy.

What percentages of nodules are malignant?

5–6% of nodules.

What are the factors which can be indicative of possible malignancy?

- Ages below 20 and above 60 years
- Men

- Previous irradiation
- Previous history of Hashimoto's disease
- Family history of MEN 2a and 2b
- History of swelling rapidly increasing in size
- History of pressure symptoms on esophagus, trachea, recurrent laryngeal nerve
- Presence of palpable neck nodes
- Ultrasound showing hypoechoic solid nodules, hypervascularity, microcalcification and capsular invasion
- FNAC shows signs of malignancy
- Thyroid-stimulating hormone (TSH) increase.

Will you suggest any medical treatment to your patient?

Radioactive ^{131}I can reduce the volume of goiter by 40% after a single dose. Prior to ^{131}I, recombinant TSH is given to stimulate greater uptake of ^{131}I.

Does suppression of TSH help?

The level of T_4 necessary to suppress TSH can cause atrial fibrillation and osteoporosis. Moreover, once T_4 is stopped, goiter increases in size again.

Which is the preferred surgical procedure?

Near total thyroidectomy; this involves total lobectomy and isthmusectomy with more than 90% of the contralateral lobe being removed.

This preserves thyroid tissue and hence T_4 replacement may not be needed. Parathyroids on one side are preserved and so hypoparathyroidism is avoided. The parathyroid gland has a caramel color because of the adipose tissue around it.

If recurrence occurs, then only one tracheoesophageal groove area has to be operated on, whereas in subtotal thyroidectomy both tracheoesophageal grooves can be involved increasing morbidity due to nerve injury.

What are the complications of ^{131}I ablation?

1. Radiation thyroiditis is not very common.
2. Hyperthyrodism may be transient. It is due to TSH receptor antibodies.
3. Hypothyroidism can also be transient.
4. Sometimes goiter increases in size initially and can worsen pressure symptoms such as stridor.

What are thyroid incidentomas and thyroid microcarcinomas?

Thyroid microcarcinoma is a papillary carcinoma less than 1.5 cm (median 8 mm).

Incidentomas are nodules which occur frequently and are not noticed. They are usually less than 1 cm and not likely to be malignant.

How will you identify the recurrent laryngeal nerve during surgery?

The recurrent laryngeal nerve bisects the angle between the inferior thyroid artery and the trachea. The recurrent laryngeal nerve lies in a triangle (Beahr's). The three sides of the triangle are—the recurrent laryngeal nerve, the carotid sheath and the inferior thyroid artery.

What is a non-recurrent laryngeal nerve?

0.5% of right recurrent laryngeal nerves are non-recurrent.

How do you identify the superior laryngeal nerve?

The superior laryngeal nerve lies in the Joll's triangle, which is bounded laterally by the upper pole of the thyroid gland, superiorly by the attachment of the strap muscles to the thyroid cartilage and medially by the midline. The floor is formed by the cricothyroid muscle.

What are the anatomical variations of the superior laryngeal nerve?

Type 1 nerve is more than 1 cm from the upper pole and hence not likely to be injured.

Type 2a nerve is within 1 cm of the upper pole whereas type 2b crosses on the surface of the thyroid. Type 2a and 2b are at risk during surgery.

If thyroid surgery is done when T_4 is raised, what complications can follow thyroid surgery?

Thyroid storm.

How do you manage it?

Thyroid storm is a potentially life-threatening condition with features of extreme hyperthyroidism. The hyperpyrexia, atrial fibrillation and probable multiorgan failure is best treated in ICU.

What are the complications of thyroidectomy?

Early complications:

1. Hemorrhage normally occurs within the first 24 hours after surgery (reactionary hemorrhage). Patient has to be re-anesthetized and bleeding looked for from the inferior thyroid veins or inferior thyroid artery (triangle of concern). Hemorrhage can also result in stridor due to supraglottic edema.
2. Voice change may be due to involvement of recurrent or superior laryngeal nerves. The nerve may have been stretched, included in a ligature, divided and injured by cauterization. So, palsy may be transient or permanent.
3. Respiratory obstruction—large goiter may have caused maleic trachea.

The trachea was held open by the mass. On removal of the mass, the trachea collapses to cause respiratory obstruction. Needs endotracheal intubation or tracheostomy.

4. Temporary hypoparathyroidism due to ischemia of the parathyroid glands.

Intermediate complications:

1. Infections.
2. Temporary palsy of recurrent or superior laryngeal nerves (less than 2%).

Late complications:

1. Subclinical hypothyroidism.
2. Permanent hypothyroidism.
3. Permanent paralysis of recurrent or superior laryngeal nerves.

What is extracapsular dissection of thyroid gland?

This allows for preservation of the parathyroid gland which can later be transplanted into the sternomastoid muscle. It also reduces risk of injury to the recurrent laryngeal nerve.

What is Berry's ligament?

The thyroid gland is attached to the trachea on its posterior surface by a condensation of fascia called Berry's ligament. The middle thyroid veins are found here and the ligament has to be resected by sharp dissection.

What is Loop of Galen?

The recurrent laryngeal nerve divides into 2 or 3 branches before entering the larynx. One of these branches is sensory. These terminal branches of the recurrent laryngeal nerve form a loop with the terminal branches of the superior laryngeal nerve; and this is called the loop of Galen.

What is Tubercle of Zuckerkandl?

This is a posterior or lateral extension of the thyroid lobe. It represents the point of fusion of ultimobranchial body with the medial anlage. The recurrent laryngeal nerve is medial to it and the tubercle of Zuckerkandl may be left behind inadvertently during surgery.

What is the cause of asymmetry of two recurrent laryngeal nerves?

Left recurrent laryngeal nerve has to ascend from the thorax because the sixth arch persists till birth as ligamentum arteriosum.

Why is right recurrent laryngeal nerve sometimes not recurrent?

Right recurrent laryngeal nerve is not recurrent when right subclavian artery arises from the dorsal aortic arch and passes to the right, posterior to the esophagus. The left recurrent laryngeal nerve can also be nonrecurrent and the right recurrent laryngeal nerve can ascend from the thorax if there is a right sided aortic arch and hence the ligamentum arteriosum is on the right side.

What are the other forms of thyroid surgery?

Miccoli technique for minimally invasive thyroid surgery:
A 15–20 mm central neck incision is made. 3–4 units of CO_2 is insufflated to create an operative pocket. A 5 mm 30 degrees high resolution endoscope is used for resection. This can be employed even for malignant diseases. Laryngeal nerve monitoring can be used as adjuvant.

Robotic thyroidectomy:
Transaxillary robotic thyroidectomy eliminates neck incision. da Vinci surgical system is used. 3-dimensional environment is created with 30 degrees optics. This improves visualization. Surgeon can control endoscope and three instruments at a time. The disadvantage is that there is no tactile feedback to the surgeon.

A vertical line is marked in the neck from hyoid to suprasternal notch. An incision is made in the axilla. A line is drawn from the superior aspect of the incision in the axilla to the upper end of the line drawn in the neck. Another line is drawn from the inferior end of the axillary incision to the inferior end of the line in the neck. Another incision of about 8 mm is made in the ipsilateral chest near the nipple for the fourth robotic arm. The thyroidectomy is done by proceeding from the axilla to the neck. Once space is created in the neck, the arm of the da Vinci system is oriented to insert the instruments. Harmonic shears are used to dissect upper and lower pole of the thyroid gland. The downside is that this is not cost-effective.

Chapter 21

Thyroglossal Cyst

A 12-year-old male presents with a swelling in the midline of the neck—4 years.

HISTORY OF PRESENT ILLNESS

It started as a small swelling of the size of a peanut and grew to its present size of a lemon over the past two years.

All questions as in chapter 19.

Examination of the neck reveals a mass 2.5 cm x 2.5 cm in the midline of the neck at the level of the hyoid bone. It is circular in shape. The skin over the swelling is normal. There is no other fistula or swelling present. The swelling moves with deglutition. It also moves when the tongue is protruded.

Palpation reveals a smooth cystic mass, which is fluctuant, non-transilluminant and not compressible. The edges of the swelling are palpable. *(Edge does not slip as it does in benign tumors such as lipoma).*

It is 2.5 cm x 2.5 cm in size.

No engorged vessels seen over the swelling. It is not pulsatile (swelling over a vessel or arising from a vessel are pulsatile; e.g. carotid body tumors).

The size of the swelling does not increase or decrease during respiration *(laryngocele).*

No other swelling palpable in the neck. The architecture of the larynx and trachea is normal. Carotid pulsations are felt on both sides.

Oral cavity and oropharynx are normal.

Indirect laryngoscopy: Posterior third of the tongue is normal; no other abnormality seen.

Diagnosis: Thyroglossal cyst.

Differential diagnosis:

1. Swelling of thyroid isthmus; soft/firm swelling.
2. Subhyoid bursitis also soft, moves on protruding tongue.
3. Pretracheal/laryngeal lymph node may be soft, firm or hard but not likely to be cystic.

Can it be a branchial cyst?

This is usually seen along the anterior border of sternomastoid muscle.

Name some lateral neck swellings?

See list given in chapter 19.

Is thyroglossal cyst always in the midline?

Sometimes it can be to the left.
Investigations

1. Ultrasound.
2. Aspiration may not be necessary and can cause infection. It is mostly never the only thyroid tissue, though it may well have thyroid gland tissue. Hence, isotope study is not necessary.
3. Thyroid function tests.

What is a thyroglossal cyst?

Thyroid primordium develops in the floor of the mouth at the site of foramen cecum and descends through tongue tissue. It passes anterior to the hyoid bone to lie in the neck anteriorly. So, the site of origin of the thyroid gland and its position in the neck is marked by the thyroglossal duct. If this duct does not involute completely, it results in a thyroglossal cyst or fistula.

How will you treat this?

The operation performed is Sistrunk's operation. Through a horizontal incision, the cyst is dissected out. As the duct passes either through or posterior to the hyoid bone, hyoid body is skeletonized and removed along with the tract. The tract is followed to the tongue and if no tract is clearly visible then a core of tissue is removed up to the foramen cecum.

If histology reveals papillary carcinoma in the thyroglossal cyst, what is the management?

If there are no nodes and if thyroid gland is normal, it is enough to estimate thyroglobulin and suppress TSH. If thyroid gland is involved, particularly in young people, a total thyroidectomy should be done.

Chapter 22

Parotid Swelling

A 50-year-old man presented with a swelling on the left side of the face—6 years duration.

HISTORY OF PRESENT ILLNESS

It started as a small swelling 6 years ago, when it was the size of his finger tip and has been growing gradually in size. There is no sudden change in the size of the swelling *(sudden increase in size is usually due to malignant transformation or hemorrhage into the mass).*

The swelling is not associated with pain *(pain is a feature of acute parotitis or acute exacerbation of a chronic problem).*

Does the swelling increase in size and cause pain during mastication?

No.
This is usual in calculus or any form of obstruction to the duct. Calculus is more common in the submandibular gland as the secretions are mucoid.

Are there any other swellings or enlargement of other salivary glands?

No.
If yes, it can be due to autoimmune diseases such as Mikulicz's syndrome, Sjorgren's syndrome.

Are there any ophthalmic symptoms like dry eyes, systemic symptoms including arthalgia?

No.
This is seen in syndromes like Sjogren's.

Is there any ulcer or mass in the skin of the face?

No.
Secondaries from lesions in the skin and face can be seen in the parotid region.

Are there any symptoms of facial nerve paralysis?

No.
Facial nerve paralysis with parotid enlargement usually indicates malignancy. It can also be seen in tuberculosis of the parotid gland.

Is there a history of irradiation/exposure to radiation even if it was 15–20 years ago?

No.
Exposure to irradiation increases chances of salivary tumors mostly malignant ones but also benign tumors. Malignant, e.g. Mucoepidermoid carcinoma, Benign such as Warthin's tumor and even pleomorphic adenoma.

Is there a history of cigarette smoking?

No.
Cigarette smoking increase chances of Warthin's tumor.

Hormonal influence and diets high in polysaturated fatty acids are seen as etiological factors for parotid tumors (malignant). Occupation of the patient (Silica dust, rubber workers, exposure to nitrosamines) can cause malignant salivary gland tumors.

From the history what is your diagnosis?

It appears to be benign mass in the parotid.

Can it be malignant?

Symptoms of neural involvement (VII cranial nerve) is not seen. It has been slow growing over a long period (6 years) There is no sudden increase in size.

Can it be an inflammatory swelling?

There are no symptoms of pain, recurrent increase and decrease in size.

Can it be a granulomatous lesion?

One has to bear tuberculosis in mind even though it is rare.

General examination: as in all cases.

On Examination

There is a swelling about 3 cm x 4 cm in the preauricular region just below the tragus. The hollow below the lobule of the ear is obliterated. (the ear lobule is lifted upwards) the skin over the swelling is normal. There are no sinuses or fistula.

- Preauricular sinus can occur in front of the tragus
- The postaural region is normal

- On palpation—the swelling is firm in consistency, not pulsatile, margins are palpable. It measure 3 cm x 4 cm. It is not hard or tender. Skin over the swelling is mobile
- No swelling palpable in the region above the tragus
- The mobility of the swelling over the masseter was tested by asking the patient to clench the teeth (masseter contracts). It is not fixed to the masseter muscle
- Bimanual palpation does not reveal any mass
  (Finger is placed in the oral cavity behind the third molar teeth in front of the anterior pillar of tonsil, the other hand is placed behind the ramus of mandible)
  The opening of the parotid duct opposite the second upper molar tooth is normal. No pus or blood is expressed at the opening of the duct on gently massaging the parotid
- *The terminal part of the duct can be palpated by inserting the index finger into the oral cavity and the thumb over the cheek)*
- No thickening of duct or calculi palpated. There is not fistula in relation to the duct or parotid gland
- Palpation of right preauricular region does not reveal any mass
  (Bilateral parotid involvement can occur in parotitis as well as in Warthin's)
  Other salivary glands are not palpable
  (Multiple salivary gland involvement is seen in autoimmune diseases)
- Facial nerve function is normal. V Cranial nerve is normal
- Examination of nodes in the preauricular, submandibular, submental nodes. No nodes are palpable
- Examination of the neck reveals no nodal enlargement
- Examination of the skin of head and neck does not reveal any abnormality (ulcer's swellings)
- Examination of the oral cavity: NAD
- No trismus
- *Trismus is caused by involvement of temporomandibular joint or masseter muscle*
- Examination of the oropharynx, no medial displacement of the pharynx or tonsil. *(this is seen in parapharyngeal tumors)*
- Examination of larynx NAD
- Ears/nose NAD.

Is the examination of the nose/ears and larynx significant?

Some, salivary gland tumors like pleomorphic adenoma's can occur from nose to brochus, middle ear, external auditory canal and lacrimal gland.

Diagnosis: Benign parotid tumor.

What are the structures which mimic parotid enlargement?

- Hypertrophy of masseter
- Sebaceous cyst in the preauricular region

- Dental cysts
- Branchial cysts
- Neuroma of facial nerve
- Aneurysm of superficial temporal artery
- Mandibular tumor
- Preauricular lymphadenitis.

What are the benign parotid swellings?

The common ones are:
- Pleomorphic adenoma.
- Warthin's tumor
- Myoepithelioma
- Oncocytoma.

The most common is pleomorphic adenomas.
80% of pleomorphic adenomas arising from the parotid occur in the superficial lobe of parotid, 20% in the deep lobe. 11% are seen in submandibular gland. It can occur rarely in sublingual and minor salivary glands.

Depending on its components, it can range from soft to firm to hard in consistency if chondroid elements are present. Calcification occurs most commonly in pleomorphic adenoma.

Among all tumors arising in the major salivary glands 70% are from the parotid. 11% from the submandibular and the rest from minor salivary glands. Among the 70% tumors in the parotid three fourths are benign; of which 84% pleomorphic adenoma 12% Warthin's tumors.

The most common minor salivary gland tumor occurs in the palate and in more than half the cases it in benign.

What are the clinical signs of parotid malignancy?

- Facial nerve paralysis
- Pain
- Fixation to skin
- Regional lymph node metastasis.

How will proceed to investigate?

- Ultrasound
- MRI
- CE-CT (Contrast-enhanced CT)
- Conventional sialography
- Salivary gland scintigraphy
- FNAC
- Immune histochemistry.

1. **Ultrasound:** The normal gland is homogenous and more echogenic than muscle.
   Neoplasm is hypoechoic as compared to normal gland.

Ultrasound can delineate retromandibular vein and superficial temporal artery. It cannot delineate facial nerve.
Malignant lesions have low reflectivity with ill defined borders.

Pleomorphic adenoma has variable reflectivity with well defined margins. Inflammatory lesions have high reflectivity with diffuse borders. With color Doppler ultrasonography malignant lesion has high vascularity. Pleomorphic adenoma has peripheral vascularity with central hypovascular area.

Disadvantage of ultrasound: It cannot evaluate deep lobe mass, parapharyngeal mass, mass obscured by mandible, Ultrasound can be used to do a ultrasound guided FNAC or to drain an abscess.

2. **MRI:** With contrast/not needed for routine cases.
   Bilateral non-enhancing lesion showing microcysts likely to be Warthin's, less likely is necrotizing lymph node, lymphoepithelial cyst.

   Unilateral or bilateral non-enhancing with high T_2 weighted signal—Warthin's not likely to be branchial cyst or necrotizing node.

   Mass showing homogenous or heterogenous appearance low to intermediate T_1, weighted image and hyperintense T_2 weighted image not invading tissue planes. Could be pleomorphic adenoma.

   Intermediate to low T_2 weighted image with or without invasion of tissue planes—adenoid cystic carcinoma.

   Malignant tumors if of low grade may resemble benign ones on MRI. If it is high grade than T_2 weighted images are of low intensity, tissue planes may be invaded, bony changes and perineural involvement is seen. These are signs of malignancy.

   Deep lobe parotid tumors may spread to prestyloid compartment between stylomandibular ligament and mandible.

   Hence, it has a dumbbell shaped appearance as it passes through the narrow stylomandibular space. To distinguish between deep parotid tumors extending to parapharyngeal space and tumor from minor salivary gland in parapharyngeal space it will be seen that:
   - Deep lobe tumor is connected to the superficial lobe at least in some sections
   - The parapharyngeal fat is displaced medially in deep lobe tumors
   - If tumor is in the prestyloid compartment carotid artery is pushed posteriorly whereas if tumor is in the poststyloid compartment carotid artery is pushed anteriorly. Poststyloid tumors of neurogenic origin have a uniform enhancement where as glomus has a salt and pepper appearance.
     MRI is not good for inflammatory lesions.
3. **CT/CE-CT:** It is the best imaging for calculi. It also differentiates between solid and cystic lesions. It can differentiate between deep lobe tumor and parapharyngeal tumor. Low density fat between parotid and constric-

tor muscle is pushed medially by deep lobe tumor and laterally by parapharyngeal tumor.
It can differentiate lymphoma from other neoplastic lesions.

It differentiates between intrinsic and extrinsic pathology of salivary glands for example, a node superficial to the submandibular gland from the submandibular gland or a sebaceous cyst outside the parotid gland.

CT with contrast is better than CT Sialography. CT Sialography was used when CT was not good.

4. **Sialography:** It is good for depicting extra and intraglandular ducts. Disadvantages are it cannot flow beyond obstruction. Sometimes it is difficult to cannulate the sub-mandibular duct. It can also cause bleeding, traumatic rupture of duct. It cannot to done in acute sialadenitis, contrast allergy, thyroid disease.
5. **Salivary gland scintigraphy:** It can be done in functional patents. It is non-invasive, low radiation. Intravenous Injection of ^{99}TC—Pertechnetate is given and salivary glands are stimulated with lemon stick 15 minutes after injecting the radionuclide.
6. **Fine needle aspiration cytology:** It has 80–90% accuracy in differentiating benign from malignant masses. Sensitivity 85.5 to 99% specificity 96.3 to 100%.
   Some problems are:
   - It cannot distinguish between Basal Cell adenoma/adenoid cystic Carcinoma
   - Mucoepidermoid carcinoma cytologically mimics salivary duct obstruction
   - FNAC is necessary to avoid resecting lymphoma's and inflammatory lesions and to avoid extensive surgery in the elderly
   - FNAC can cause seeding of tumor cells. To avoid this 25 gauge needle can be used. This prevents tumor infarction and seeding.
7. **Immune histochemistry:** It is useful for looking for locoregional recurrence and for prognosis. It is still not very useful diagnostically.

   Proliferative cell nuclear antigen (PCNA) is increased in malignant cells as compared to benign tumors. K1-67 is an antibody which binds to an antigen in a dividing cell. So the proportion of K1-67 gives an indication of how many cells are proliferating.

- K1-67 index is < 5% in benign tumors
- K1-67 index is > 10% malignant tumors.

It is also useful in the prognosis of adenoid cystic carcinoma.

BCl_2 inhibits apoptosis. It can be a useful prognostic marker.
Cytokeratin 14 is a marker for squamous cell carcinoma. It is also raised in myoepithelial tumors.

Fibroblast growth factor 1 and 2 and fibroblast growth factor receptor 1 is increased in malignant salivary tumor.

Mucin type carbohydrate antigen Sialyl T_n is associated with locoregional recurrence.

Estrogen and progesterone receptors are seen more frequently in malignant tumors and can be of therapeutic value.

What is a Warthin's Tumor?

This occurs only in the parotid because rest of the salivary glands do not have lymphoid tissue. It is seen in the lower lobe in the seventh decade of life. It is a soft swelling and may have microcysts in the mass. It is frequently bilateral. It has a eosinophilic glandular epithelium with stroma of lymphocytes, which can form follicles or cysts. It can arise along with other parotid tumors especially pleomorphic adenoma.

What are the other common salivary tumors?

Myoepithelioma has solely myoepithelial cells. It may be a variant of pleomorphic adenoma.

Oncocytoma: Common in parotid and is seen in the 7–8th decade. It is benign and excision is sufficient.

What are the inflammatory lesions of the parotid gland?

If there are only local symptoms of inflammation, it can be viral or bacterial. Common viral infection is mumps causing bilateral parotitis. Infection is self limiting.

Bacterial infection may lead to formation of pus below the capsule of the parotid. So drainage can only occur after elevating a skin flap. Ultrasound guided needle aspiration of pus can be done.

If there is a chronic enlargement of the parotid with recurrent acute exacerbation then there may be ductal block which has to be evaluated by X-ray or CT. This has to be followed by dilatation sialoplasty. If no obstruction is present immunological evaluation has to be done.

Other non-neoplastic causes can be Sjogren's syndrome and tuberculosis.

How does tuberculosis involve the parotid gland?

It can spread via the tonsil, to the parotid duct or by hematogenous spread from the lungs. It can present as an acute sialadenitis or a chromic enlargement of the parotid. There may be no constitutional symptoms.

How does HIV involve the salivary glands?

This is frequent and may be the first indication of the viral infection. There is lymphocytic proliferation, lymphoid tissue hypertrophy and cystic lesions in the gland.

If FNAC and other investigations reveal that the mass is a pleomorphic adenoma, how will you proceed?

If the lesion is limited to the superficial part, then I will do a superficial parotidectomy.

Why not simply remove the mass?

Pleomorphic adenoma does not have a complete capsule and so some tissue may be left back if only mass is removed. This can result in recurrent pleomorphic adenoma which may be multiple and so more difficult to dissect. Pleomorphic adenoma left behind can also recur as carcinoma in pleomorphic adenoma and this has a bad prognosis.

Describe the incision for superficial parotidectomy

It is a lazy S incision starting from in front of the tragus and curves around the lobule of the ear going backwards up to the mastoid tip and extending horizontally in the neck to the hyoid bone. The incision is superficial in the face and subplatysmal in the neck.

How will you Identify the Facial Nerve?

During surgery the following landmarks can be used:

a. The tragal point; the tragal cartilage ends in a point and the facial nerve is 1 cm below and deep to it.
b. It can also be traced where the posterior belly of digastric muscle attaches to the mastoid process. It is immediately above the attachment at its anterior border (of the muscle).
c. The junction between the cartilaginous and bony external canal wall. The nerve lies immediately deep and inferior to it.
d. To trace one of the peripheral braches to the main trunk. It is better to trace the buccal branch which runs parallel to and 1 cm below the arch of the zygoma. It is better not to trace the marginal mandibular because accidental injury gives rise to a visible deformity. Always use facial nerve monitor.

What are the complications of parotidectomy?

1. Facial nerve weakness/palsy. If cut, then an end to end anastomosis or a nerve graft has to be done (All details of facial nerve injury refer to ear surgery)
2. Frey's syndrome:

   It is the gustatory sweating that occurs on the face during mastication. The auriculotemporal nerve provides parasympathetic innervation to the parotid gland and when transaction of the nerve occurs during parotidectomy the cut end of the nerve develops new axons which supplies the sweat glands of the face. So sweating occurs on that side of the face during mastication. The most effective treatment is injection of botulinum type A toxin.

   Treatment:

   a. Reassurance
   b. Topical anticholinergics
   c. Resection of Jacobson's nerve over the promontory in the middle ear.

   d. Interposition of fascia or fat between secretomotor fibers and skin.
   e. Stellate ganglion block.
   f. Injection of botulinum type A toxin
3. Numbness of ear flowing resection of greater auricular nerve.
4. Parotid fistula, rare and self-limiting.

What are the types of parotidectomy?

1. Superficial parotidectomy—superficial lobe is removed.
2. Total conservative—superficial + deep lobe removed
3. Total radical—superficial + deep lobe + facial nerve.
4. Extended radical parotidectomy—total radical + contiguous structures such as ramus of mandible/Zygomatic arch/temporalis and sternomastoid muscles/bony and cartilaginous external auditory canal/mastoid, etc.

What are the theories of salivary gland neoplasia?

Multicellular theory: Each type arises from different cell in the salivary gland this is because all the cells retain the capacity for mitoses and regeneration. According to this theory Warthin's tumor and oncocytic tumor arise from striated ductal cell, acinar from acinar cell, mixed parotid tumor from myoepithehal and intercalated duct.

Bicellular theory: According to this theory tumor arises from basal cells of excretory or intercalated duct. This theory believes that these two cell types can differentiate into all other cells. Adenomatous tumor such as pleomorphic adenoma arises from intercalated cells whereas squamous cell carcinoma and mucoepidermoid carcinoma arise from excretory duct cells.

The persistence of neuroectodermal antigen in both benign and malignant tumor has led to a single stem cell origin of tumor (neuroectodermal cell) As salivary tumor have many cell types it can be explained by its origin from a single pluripotent cell.

Chapter 23

Submandibular Gland Swelling

A 50-year-old woman presents with a swelling below the jaw on the right side—2 months' duration.

HISTORY OF PRESENT ILLNESS

Swelling was small to start with, size of a grape. It has gradually progressed to the present size (of a lemon).

Swelling is associated with pain.

Pain is dull aching not related to food and swelling does not increase in size during mastication.

(Pain/increase in size during mastication is characteristic of calculi).

Size increases because calculi prevents secretions from reaching oral cavity.

Is there any abnormality of tongue movement?

No.

Salivary gland tumors can involve hypoglossal nerve.

Are there any other swellings in the neck?

No.

Mikulicz syndrome results in multiple salivary gland involvement.

Is there deviation of angle of the mouth?

No.

This is due to involvement of marginal mandibular nerve.

(Rest of the questions same as in chapter 22).

From the history what is your diagnosis?

- It may be a submandibular gland swelling or a lymph node
- Appears to be a new growth, as there are no symptoms of inflammation
- Swelling is associated with pain may be malignant.

General Examination: As in all other cases.

On examination: There is a swelling visible below the middle third of the lower margin of the mandible on the right side. It is about 5 cm in greatest dimension ovoid in shape, skin over the swelling is normal, the swelling is not pulsatile, no sinus or fistula seen over the swelling. The swelling is partly below the inferior margin of the mandible.

On palpation, it is firm in consistency, not tender, 4 cm in size, upper limit of the swelling is palpable below the inferior margin of the mandible. It does not cross the midline anteriorly and is above the level of the hyoid bone. The inferior margin of the mandible is free. The swelling moves in all directions. No pulsations felt. It is firm in consistency.

Bimanual palpation:
One finger of one hand is placed on the floor of the mouth medial to the alveolus and lateral to the tongue and pressed on the floor of the mouth. The finger of the other hand is placed just medial to the inferior margin of the mandible. This finger is pushed upwards. This helps to palpate both deep and superficial lobes.
The swelling is bimanually palpable.
(Lymph nodes are not bimanually palpable as they lie out side the mylohyoid muscle completely)
No other stone or calculus felt.

The Wharton's duct opening at the floor of the mouth on either side of the frenulum linguae, shows no signs of inflammation. Protrusion of the tongue and tongue movements are normal.

- Facial nerve is normal (no deviation of the angle of the mouth)
- No other palpable swelling in the face or neck
- Oral cavity/oropharynx/larynx/ear/nose and PNS are normal.

Diagnosis: Benign/malignant swelling of the submandibular salivary gland right side.

No definite signs of malignancy such as nerve involvement/skin involvement/nodes, etc.

What is the commonest benign swelling of the submandibular gland?

Pleomorphic adenoma.

What are the common malignant tumors of the submandibular salivary gland?

- Adenoid cystic carcinoma—43%
- Mucoepidermoid carcinoma—17%
- Adenocarcinoma—11%.

What is the common malignant tumor of parotid gland?

Mucoepidermoid carcinoma followed by adenoid cystic carcinoma.

What do you know about these malignant tumors?

1. Adenoid cystic carcinoma—common sites are submandibular, parotid and palate. 70% have pulmonary metastasis at presentation but these double slowly. It is blood borne.

- Adenoid cystic carcinoma is of three types histologically
- Solid—40% (worse prognosis)
- Cribiform—25% (better prognosis)
- Tubular—20% (better prognosis)
- There is 100% recurrence at primary site at 30 years.
- It spreads perineurally (80%)
- If it a large tumor with perineural spread—radical resection of primary + nerve excision + chemo RT is the treatment
- Small tumor—radical excision of mass ± irradiation.

2. Mucoepidermoid carcinoma:
   It involves the major salivary glands can be a painless mass or cause painful swelling with relevant nerve involvement. It used to be divided as low, intermediate and high grade but is now classified either as low or high grade.
   - It has mucous secreting cells, epidermoid cells and intermediate cells
   - Low grade tumors are cystic
   - High grade tumors are solid with 75% having a neck node metastasis
   - It is supposed to arise from the intercalated duct reserve cell (common progenitor cell).

   Treatment (when it involves the parotid)
   - Low grade tumors—superficial parotidectomy with facial nerve preservation
   - High grade tumors—radical excision + neck dissection of 1, 2, 3 levels with RT to regional area and neck
   - If neck nodes are present—radical excision + radical neck dissection + RT to local area and neck
3. Adenocarcinoma—it has ductal and tubular formation Histological grading according to mitosis, cellular pleomorphism and stromal invasion. This decides whether it is low or high grade. Better to regard all as high grade. Most common in the parotid.

What are the other malignant tumors you know?

1. Acinar cell carcinoma can sometimes be bilateral, usually seen in the parotid as a painless lump. Can histologically resemble many salivary and non-salivary tumors like mucoepidermoid carcinoma, myoepithelial carcinoma, oncocytoma, metastatic renal disease, thyroid cancer, etc.
   - Good prognosis
   - Treatment is surgery, sparing VII N with neck dissection + postoperative radiotherapy.
2. Polymorphic low grade carcinoma—it is a low grade variant of adenoid cystic carcinoma. Benign course, local excision is adequate.
3. Carcinoma ex pleomorphic adenoma occurs most commonly in recurrent pleomorphic adenoma. If there is malignant transformation in men over 40 years with deep lobe involvement the prognosis is bad. Depth of invasion of more than 1 cm is associated with bad prognosis.

Histologically, it can be a carcinoma, carcinosarcoma, metastizing mixed tumor or non-invasive carcinoma. Same tumor can have malignant and benign elements.

- Prognosis is poor.

4. Squamous cell carcinoma—for a salivary gland tumor to be called squamous cell carcinoma.
   - It must arise from gland not from lymph node
   - No primary should be detected in the skin or adjacent structures
   - High grade mucoepidermoid carcinoma should be excluded.

   It is common in the parotid. Facial palsy may be present. Neck nodes are positive in 50% of cases at presentation facial paralysis and neck nodes denote poor prognosis.
5. Undifferentiated carcinoma—in this tumor (Epstein-Barr virus) EBV may have a role. This resembles small cell nasopharyngeal cancer. Irradiation is the best modality.
6. Lymphoma—Sjogren's syndrome may develop into lymphoma.
   3 criteria to classify tumor as lymphoma are:
   - Extraglandular lymphoma must not be present
   - Must be from glandular parenchyma not from intraglandular lymph node
   - Immunohitischemistry (IHC) must confirm diagnosis
     Treatment is chemotherapy.

What tumors metastasize to the parotid?

- Skin tumor mostly posterior to the facial artery (includes pinna and lacrimal gland
- Lung, breast and renal tumor can metastazise to parotid.

How will you investigate the case?

As in chapter 22 + CT/MRI of lung, bone and liver.

How will you treat?

- If is a pleomorphic adenoma—submadibular gland excision
- If it is adenoid cystic carcinoma—remove whole submandibular gland and since it is N_0, level 1, 2, 3 nodes resection
- If other than N_0 (N_1 to N_3): radical neck dissection
- If nerve is positive—resection of nerve.

What is the incision for submandibular gland resection?

Incision is parallel to a natural skin crease 2.5 cm below lower border of mandible and extending 10 cm from anterior border of the sternomastoid muscle.

How do you avoid injury to the marginal mandibular nerve?

- Make an incision onto the capsule and retract capsule superiorly
- Identify anterior facial vein as nerve crosses anterior facial vein. The vein is divided well below the nerve and retracted upwards so nerve is safe.

How do you approach the deep part?

Retract mylohyoid muscle medially and the deep part is seen lying over the hyoglossus muscle. Small nerve fibers from the lingual nerve to the gland (parasympathetic secretomotor fibers) have to be resected to free the lingual nerve. Hypoglossal nerve lies parallel to lingual and is superior to it. The gland is removed after duct ligation.

What are the complications?

- Marginal mandibular nerve injury
- Lingual nerve injury
- Hypoglossal nerve injury.

How will you treat recurrent pleomorphic adenoma?

- As incidence of malignant change is great imaging is followed by removal of all gland tissue
- Facial nerve monitoring is a must.

What is the TNM Classification for salivary gland tumors?

- T_1: 2 cm without extraparenchymal disease (extraparenchymal means clinical involvement of soft tissues)
- T_2: 2 to 4 cm without extraparenchymal disease
- T_3: 4–6 cm and or extraparenchymal spread
- T_4: >6 cm and or base skull/VII N involvement (any neural)
- N_1: < 3 cm single node in greatest dimension
- N_2:
- N_{2a}: 3–6 cm single same side
- N_{2b}: 3–6 cm multiple unilateral (same side)
- N_{2c}: 3–6 cm multiple bilateral or contralateral
- N_3: More than 6 cm in greatest dimension.

Staging:

- Stage I: $T_1 N_0 M_0$
- Stage II: $T_2 N_0 M_0$
- Stage III: $T_3 N_0 M_0$
$T_3 N_1 M_0$
$T_1 N_1 M_0$
$T_2 N_1 M_0$
- Stage IV A: $T_{4a} N_0 M_0$
$T_{4a} N_1 M_0$
T_1
T_2 $N_2 M_0$
T_3
$T_{4a} N_2 M_0$

- Stage IV B: T_{4b} any N M
  Any T N_3 M_0
- Stage IV C: Any T any N M_1
- T_{4a}: Moderately advanced disease tumor invades mandible/skin/ear canal/facial nerve
- T_{4b}: Very advanced disease
  Tumur invades skull base/pterygoid plates and/or encases carotid artery.

Chapter 24

Cervical Lymphadenopathy with Unknown Primary

A 45-year-old man presents with a swelling on the left side of neck—3 months duration.

HISTORY OF PRESENT ILLNESS

- It started as a small swelling, gradually increasing in size (of a small lemon)
- No history of pain

Pain is present in inflammatory process or when there is a neural involvement in malignancies

- No history of trauma
- No history of evening rise of temperature, lose of weight and appetite or cough with blood stained sputum

These symptoms are usually seen in tuberculosis. Loss of weight is also seen in malignancies

- No history of dysphagia/regurgitation of undigested food
- Dysphasia is seen in malignancy of upper gastrointestinal tract

Dysphagia and regurgitation of undigested food can occur in pharyngeal pouch

- Swelling does not alter with respiratory cycle

This occurs in laryngocele

- No history of nasal block, epistaxis, unexplained falling of teeth and trismus

These are symptoms of nose, PNS and nasopharyngeal malignancies

- No history of excision, irradiation of any mass in the head and neck or body

This history is necessary to arrive at a diagnosis of secondary node due to Head and Neck malignancies or malignancies below clavicle

- No history of ear symptoms or hearing loss or otalgia

This is seen in otitis media with effusion due to nasopharyngeal malignancies or referred pain in the ear due to nasopharyngeal and hypopharyngeal malignancies

- No symptoms of hypo or hyperthyroidism
- *A neck mass may be thyroid in origin.*

Past History
No history of tuberculosis, diabetes, or hypertension.

Family History
Not significant.

Personal History
Patient is a smoker, smoker 2 packets of beedies per day for 15 years, not an alcoholic.

Diagnosis after history:
- *Patient indicates a position of a lateral neck mass. It is of 3 months duration hence not an acute lesion*
- *No constitutional symptoms of tuberculosis. No symptoms of any primary in the head and neck region*
- *Patient is a smoker*
- *Patient is 45 years of age hence congenital and developmental masses are not likely*
- *Chronic lymph node involvement may be tuberculosis or a secondary in a lymph node.*

General Examination

Local examination
A hard single swelling in the region of the middle third of the sternomastoid on the left side. Skin over the swelling is normal. Swelling is not pulsatile.
Pulsatile swelling can be a carotid paraganglioma
Swelling does not move with deglutition or on swallowing.
Site of the swelling is important as a swelling along the sternomastoid muscle anterior border (when the upper third meets the lower two thirds of the muscle) is likely to be a branchial cyst.
More than one swelling indicates lymph node swellings.

Palpation—the swelling is 4 cm in its greatest dimension, it is oval in shape. The swelling appears to be partially beneath the sternomastoid muscle.

Relation of swelling to sternomastoid muscle can be verified by doing the following test. Place your hand on the chin of the patient opposite to the swelling and ask him to press against your hand. The sternomastoid becomes taut.

Almost all swelling in the neck are deep to the sternomastoid muscle except sternomastoid tumors. This occurs in infants and is due to birth trauma. It is an oval swelling and occurs in the middle third of the sternomastoid muscle. It is self limiting and heals by fibrosis.

- *To make both sternomastoid muscles taut place your hand at the point of the chin and ask the patient to press downwards*
- The skin over the swelling is normal and pinchable
- Swelling is hard in consistency.

Tuberculosis lymph nodes are matted due to perilymphadenitis and adherence of one node to another. It can liquefy later to form a cold abscess.

Branchial cysts are cystic in consistency.

- Swelling does not exhibit expansile pulsation (aneurysm of a vessel) or transmitted pulsation (mass lying over carotid)
- Swelling is not compressible (laryngocele), it is not transilluminant *(cysts are transilluminant)*
- Larynx appears normal
- Trachea is in the mind line
- Bocca's sign is negative.

To palpate for neck nodes:
Stand behind the patient and flex his head slightly. Place index fingers over both mastoid processes and proceed along the anterior border of the trapezius muscle till the clavicle is reached. Insert fingers along anterior border of trapezius with thumb pressing the shoulder blades forward. On reaching the clavicle posterior triangle is palpated. Nodes here lie between skin and muscles of the floor of the posterior triangle. Relax the sternomastoid muscle by pushing the patients head towards the examined side. Curve fingers and proceed in front of the sternomastoid anterior border with thumb behind the muscle. A 'C' is formed on the muscle. Examine for level II, III and IV nodes Jugulodigastric muscle may be palpable in normal persons. Next go along the suprasternal notch and palpate midline of neck (Level VI), Following this the submental and submandibular nodes and preauricular modes can be palpated.

Structures mistaken for nodes are:

1. Carotid bulb
2. Obstructed submandicular gland may resemble a node
3. Greater cornu of hyoid bone
4. Lateral tip of transverse process of C_1, C_2
5. Parotid Tail
6. Superior horn of thyroid cartilage.

- Examination of the nose and PNS—NAD
- Examination of the nasopharynx—NAD
- Examination of the oral cavity/oropharynx—NAD
- Palpation of posterior third of tongue and tonsil—no induration felt
- Indirect laryngoscopy—both cords normal in structure and mobility. No abnormal mass seen
- No palpable thyroid mass
- Examination of the ear—NAD
- Examination of skin of head and neck and scalp—no mass seen
- No palpable parotid or submandibular gland.

Diagnosis—Secondary neck node where the primary has not been made out on clinical examination

- $T_x N_2 M_0$
- If the primary is squamous cell carcinoma of head and neck except thyroid where it would be N_{1b} and nasopharynx when it would be N_1

What can the differential diagnoses be?

This is a swelling in the anterior triangle of the neck in a person in the 4th decade of life.

The probably causes could be

1. Tuberculosis lymphadenitis
2. Branchial cyst
3. Paraganglioma
4. Bronchogenic carcinoma.

1. Tuberculous lymphadenitis is not the first diagnosis because there are no constitutional symptoms which is seen in 50% of patients and the nodes are not matted and the node is hard. Tuberculosis cervical lymphadenitis has about 20% association with pulmonary tuberculosis. Matting of lymph nodes is due to periadenitis. Later, it can caseate and form a fistula. In India, tuberculosis has always to be borne in mind.
2. Branchial cyst usually is seen along the anterior border of the sternomastoid muscle at the junction of the upper third with the lower two thirds. It usually presents in young adults and a branchial cyst as a diagnosis in the 4th decade has to be viewed with caution lest a secondary be missed. The three, theories of origin of a branchial cyst are:
   a. Origin from a branchial pouch
   b. Origin from cervical sinus
   c. Origin from lymph node degeneration.
3. Paraganglionomas are seen in the third decade but may be considered here. It is a neural crest origin tumor. It can occur on the carotid body, vagal ganglia and jugulo tympanum. Swelling is mobile only side to side and not superior to inferior. Malignant paraganglioma are difficult to distinguish from benign on histopathological examination.
4. Branchiogenic carcinoma occurs along the line from the front of tragus to clavicle along the anterior border of sternomastoid histopathological examination should confirm carcinoma in the lining of the cyst and show branchial vestiges. Such a diagnosis can only be made if no primary is found.

Investigations:

1. X-ray chest to rule out—
   a. Primary
   b. Secondary
   c. Concomitant tuberculosis
   d. Chronic obstructive pulmonary diseases
   e. Mediastinal node.
2. CT with contrast—skull base to thoracic inlet.
   CT is particularly needed for retropharyngeal node
   If node is more than 1 cm on CT, it is a metastatic node
   Metastatic nodes on CT show, rim enhancement, central necrosis, and spherical shape.
3. MRI with Gladolinium contrast.

Shows areas of mucosal thickening, altered attenuation and asymmetry in mucosal lining which can all help to point at areas where biopsy can be taken. Both CT and MRI along with PET/CT may allow a primary to show up, 40% of the times. Of these 80% are likely to be from base tongue or tonsil.
All imagining should be done prior to biopsy to avoid artifacts.

4. PET/CT with 18 fluorodeoxyglucose helps to detect primary by indicating areas of increased metabolism.
5. Epstein-Barr virus detected directs suspicion to nasopharynx.
6. Human Papillomavirus detection points to oropharynx particularly tonsil.
7. Examination under anesthesia—to visualize nasopharynx, larynx, oropharynx and esophagus.
   If nodes are at levels I, II, III, V then examination under anesthesia palpation of oropharynx, biopsy of clinically and radiologically suspicious sites tonsillectomy, direct laryngoscopy, esophagoscopy and nasopharyngeal examination is appropriate. If nodes are in levels IV and level V in addition to the above, an esphagoscopy, chest/abdominal and pelvic CT are needed. Tonsillectomy gives more results than random biopsy from nasopharynx and posterior third of tongue.
8. Fine needle aspiration cytology of node may reveal
   a. Squamous cell carcinoma
   b. Adenocarcinoma
   c. Lymphoma
   d. Mucosal melanoma.

When microsatellite identification is done some characteristics of the primary may be seen in the node and point to the primary such as:

- Monolayered papillary fronds with intranuclear cytoplasmic inclusions–papillary thyroid carcinoma
- Large, polygonal, keratinized cells with a low nuclear/cytoplasmic ratio are seen in oral carcinoma
- Numerous naked nuclei with marked lymphocytic infiltration are seen in nasopharyngeal carcinoma
- Open biopsy of nodes alters lymphatic channels and is hence not advisable.

Where does the common unknown primary with occult metastasis usually occur?

- Common level is level II followed by level–III
- I, IV, V are less frequent
- Majority of nodes are N_2 and it is usually unilateral.

Why is an unknown primary not seen?

- Autoimmune destruction of primary
- Spontaneous regression of primary
- Accelerated tumor progression.

What are the drainage areas for various nodal levels?

	Boundaries	*Area of drainage*
Level I A submental	Bounded by anterior belly of digastric and hyoid bone	Lower lip, floor of month lower alveolus
Level I B submandibular	Bounded by posterior belly of digastric and body of mandible	Face, nose and PNS oral cavity submandibular gland
Level II A	Nodes along upper third of internal jugular vein medial to spinal accessory nerve extending from skull base to hyoid bone	
Level II B	Nodes along upper third of internal jugular vein lateral or posterior to spinal accessory extending from skull base to hyoid bone	Oral cavity, oropharynx naso-pharynx hypopharynx supraglottic larynx
Level III	Nodes along middle third of internal jugular vein from hyoid to cricoid. Omohyoid muscle crosses internal jugular vein (IJV) here	Thyroid larynx, Hypopharynx, Cervical esophagus
Jugulo omohyoid node belongs to Level III while jugulo digastric is at the junction of Level II and Level III		
Level IV	Nodes along lower third of internal jugular vein from cricoid to clavicle	Hypopharynx, intra-abdominal organs/breast, lungs, esophagus, thyroid
Level V	Nodes between posterior border of sternomastoid and anterior border of trapezius at the lower half of spinal accessory and transverse cervical artery, nodes along spinal accessory is V A, nodes along transverse cervical artery is level V B	Nasopharynx, esophagus thyroid, oropharynx, skin of scalp and neck
Level VI	Midline of neck from thyroid to suprasternal notch between the two anterior borders of sternomastoid muscle includes pre and para-tracheal nodes, pre and perilaryn-geal nodes parathyroid nodes	Thyroid hypopharynx
Level VII	Anterior mediastinal nodes	Thyroid

These patterns of lymphatic drainage are in a non-violated neck. If even lymph node biopsy is done, then the lymphatic drainage changes.

Describe N staging

- N_0: No palpable node
- N_1: Single node 3 cm or less in greatest dimension and ipsilateral
- N_{2a}: Single ipsilateral node more that 3 cm but less than 6 cm in greatest dimension
- N_{2b}: Multiple ipsilateral nodes greater than 3 cm but not more than 6 cm in greatest dimension

- N_{2c}: Multiple bilateral or contralateral nodes more than 3 cm but not greater than 6 cm in greatest dimension
- N_3: Node more than 6 cm in greatest dimension
- N: Staging in thyroid cancer
- N_0: No node
- N_{1a}: Regional lymph node metastasis level VI
- N_{1b}: Unilateral bilateral or contralateral cervical node or superior mediastinal node
- N: Staying in nasopharynx
- N_1: Unilateral 6 cm or less in greatest dimension above supraclavicular region
- N_2: Bilateral nodes 6 cm or less above supraclarvicular region
- N_3: More than 6 cm in greatest dimension extending to supraclavicular fossa.

What are the Fallacies of N Staging?

- In supraglottic larynx, if N_1 nodes are present bilaterally it has no worse prognosis than unilateral node
- In some cases, contralateral and bilateral have a worse prognosis and should go to N_3 rather than N_{2C}
- There is no mention of levels
- There is no mention of extracapsular spread
- Immunological status of nodes is not taken into account
- If there is massive node on both sides of the neck, there is almost no chance of survival; but it has not found a place in the classification.

How does nodal metastasis occur?

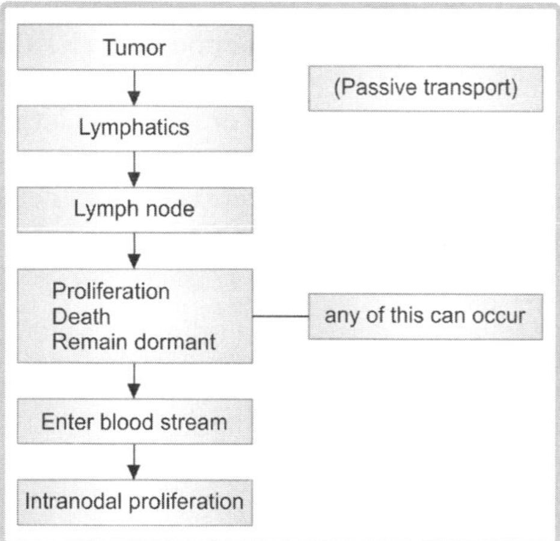

Intranodes proliferation leading to destruction of nodal architecture and progress to second echelon. Malignant cell destruction in the node may occur due to T lymphocyte sensitization leading to activation of macrophages and lymphocytes. Extracapsular invasion can occur early or late in nodal metastasis depending on how the disease spreads in the nodes.

What are the common areas that metastasize to cervical lymph nodes other than head and neck?

Lung, esophagus, renal, ovarian, cervix and prostate.

How will you treat this patient?

After all investigations:

1. If primary is found treat according to treatment of primary with neck secondries.
2. If primary is not found and if the FNAC shows squamous cell carcinoma then the following can be tried:
   a. Surgery—neck dissection and if there is no extracapsular spread CTRT has to be given as it is a N_2 node. If there is extracapsular spread then CTRT + RT to relevant mucosal area in this case–oropharynx.
   b. CTRT or RT or induction chemotheraphy can be tried instead of surgery. If following any one of these modalities the clinical response is good only follow up is needed. However, if during follow up there are positive nodes then neck dissection is needed.

What are the general guidelines for treatment of neck secondaries with occult primary?

General guidelines of treatment of neck secondaries with occult primary post neck dissection:

- N_1 with no extracapsular spread radiotherapy to neck alone or added relevant mucosal irradiation can be done
- In N_2 N_3 with no extra capsular spread chemotherapy RT can be added
- In N_2 N_3 with extra capsular spread chemotherapy RT + RT to relevant mucosal area
- If the FNAC report is adenocarcinoma and this is a level II node treatment would be neck dissection with parotidectomy (Level I–III this is the treatment)
- If FNAC is adenocarcinoma with Level IV–V node then neck dissection + evaluate infraclavicular area for primary

If the FNAC report is mucosal melanoma:

- Nodal site requires a neck dissection ± adjuvant systemic treatment

If the FNAC report is thyroid:

- Appropriate treatment for thyroid malignancy
- If FNAC reveals a lymphoma an open biopsy followed by staging and relevant treatment should be instituted

Describe the neck dissection to be done here

A modified neck dissection with preservation of two non-lymphatic structures, i.e. sternomastoid muscle and spinal accessory nerve can be done here:

1. A Schobinger incision can be used.
2. Skin incision includes platsyma.

3. Avoid injury to the mandibular branch and cervical branch of facial nerve by incising the capsule of submandibular gland and retracting it upwards.
4. Retract lower end of sternocleidomastiod muscle to reach carotid sheath. Divide lower end of internal jugular vein (IJV) between 3 ligatures. If there is an accidental tear of the IJV do not clamp but use finger pressure to stop bleeding and suture tear with 6.0 ethilon. Lower end tear can cause air embolism. On the left side thoracic duct passes medial to the IJV and then medial to it and then curves to enter where IJV meets subclavian vein.
5. Next approach Chassaignac's triangle. This triangle is between longus colli and scalenus anterior muscles and their attachment to Chassaignac's tubercle or carotid tubercle of C6 with subclavian artery as the base. This is the area of the scalene nodes which should be removed and the region where the thoracic duct is present.
6. Divide omohyoid muscle at its tendon.
7. Mobilize fat pad overlying prevertebral fascia.
8. Avoid injury to brachial plexus and phrenic nerve.
9. Dissect posterior triangle along anterior border of trapezius up to mastoid tip.
10. It is easier to identify spinal accessory nerve when it is 1 cm above Erb's point, so that the nerve can be preserved.
11. Look for upper end of IJV and ligate it.
12. Next the submandibular gland has to be dissected. Retract posterior belly of digastric muscle identify and preserve hypoglossal nerve. Dissect submandibular gland. Proceed to elevate mylohyoid muscle to tie the submandibular duct.

What are the four corners of consternation in neck dissection?

1. Ligation of internal jugular vein lower end
2. Junction of lateral border of clavicle with lower edge of trapezius
3. Ligation of internal jugular vein upper end
4. Submandibular gland dissection.

What is radical neck dissection?

Removal of nodes I-V and all three non-lymphatic structures.

What is comprehensive neck dissection?

Removal of all neck nodes as in radical neck dissection with preservation or ligation of any or all of the non-lymphatic structures.

What is extended radical neck dissection?

Radical neck dissection with removal of one or more additional nodes or non-lymphatic structures such as level VI, VII, hypoglossal nerve, digastric muscle, skin, mandible, parotid, mastoid tip.

What is selective neck dissection?

This is removal of one or more group of nodes in an N_0 neck, such as supraomohyoid neck dissection, lateral neck dissection where II, III, IV are removed. (Refer chapter 13 for classification of selective neck dissection.)

What are the complications of neck dissection?

- Hemorrhage
- Wound infection
- Carotid artery rupture
- Chylous fistula
- Pneumothorax
- Nerve injury
  - Facial nerve branches
  - Hypoglossal, lingual, vagus and sympathetic trunk
  - Phrenic nerve
  - Brachial plexus
- Cerebral edema.

What are types of altered fractionation in radiotherapy?

Altered fractionation

i. Accelarated fraction 6 fractions/week 66–74 Gy to gross disease 44–64 Gy to subclinical disease.
ii. Concomitant boost accelerated RT:
72 Gy/6 weeks 1.8 Gy/fraction large field for 7 weeks
1.5 Gy boost as second daily dose during first 12 days of RT.
iii. Hyperfractionation:
81.6 Gy/7 weeks 1.2 Gy/twice daily.

In hyperfractionation more irradiation can be given causing better locoregional control; may or may not influence disease free interval. Disease free interval may be influenced in patients below 60 years.

In chemotherapy RT, it is better to give conventional fractionation.
Mucosal Dose: 50–60 Gy/2 Gy/day, consider higher dose for suspicious area.
Evaluate RT results after 12 weeks with PET/CT scan.
Complete clinical response implies:

a. No palpable nodes
b. No radiological node larger than 1.5 cm
c. Pathological confirmation.

If radiologically 1.5–2.5 cm node is present, neck dissection is necessary. CTRT is better if there is extracapsular spread or positive margins. Pan mucosal irradiation is replaced by selective mucosal irradiation depending upon level of node.

What is the prognosis in secondary metastasis with occult primary?

50%: 5 years survival rate.

INDEX

A

Abdomen 5
Abdominal surgery 118
Acanthosis 99
Acid regurgitation 118
Acinar cell carcinoma 191
Acoustic reflex 42
Acoustic rhinometry 53
Acoustic voice measurement 123
Adenocarcinoma 79, 191
Adenoid 81
 cystic carcinoma 190
Aerated middle turbinate 65
Agger nasi cell 65
Alexander's law 11, 37, 40
Allergic and non-allergic rhinitis 49
Allergic rhinitis 57
Allergies 159
Alveolar tumors 69
Amelanotic melanoma 87
Amyotrophic lateral sclerosis 127
Anaplastic carcinoma 170
Anaplastic thyroid cancer 165
Anastomotic leak 156
Aneurysm 8
 of superficial temporal artery 183
Angiofibroma, histopathology of 82
Angiosarcoma 79
Angle of mouth, deviation of 189
Anorexia 159
Anterior cranial fossa, floor of 79
Anterior ethmoidal artery, course of 62
Antral lavage 62
Antrochoanal polyp 49, 58
Antrum, large 16
Arthalgia 180
Aryepiglottic fold 120, 134
Arytenoid 120, 134
 dislocation 116
Asthma 159
Atelectatic process 8
Audiometry, absence of 10
Auditory brainstem evoke response 44
Auditory canal disease, symptoms of
 external 1
Auditory canal, external 6, 22
Auditory evoke potential 44
Aural polyp 6

B

Bad smell in the mouth 94
Basal cell
 carcinoma 70
 hyperplasia 23
Basaloid squamous cell carcinoma 146
Belfast rule of thumb 26
Bell's palsy 28, 29
Benign nasal tumors, symptoms of 67
Benign swelling in nasopharynx 81
Benign tumors 146
 classify 67
Benign ulcers of oral cavity 97
Berry's ligament 176
Bezold abscess 31
Bicellular theory 188
Bilateral ethmoidal polypi 57
Bilateral nasal polypi 51
Bilateral vocal cord paralysis 129
Blood
 dyscracias 50
 stained nasal discharge 67
Bocca's sign 86, 121, 197
Bone
 conduction 9, 45
 thickening 62
Bony orbital wall 75
Brachial plexus 204
Brachytherapy 92
Brackmann's grade correlate 30
Brain abscess 5, 31, 32
Branchial cyst 157, 183
Brun's nystagmus 11

Buccal carcinoma 99
Buccal mucosa 96
Buccinator 27
Bulla ethmoidalis, large 65

C

Cafe-au-lait spots 70
Calorie test 37
Canal infection, external 1
Canal paresis 37
Cancer larynx 130
Carcinoma 192
 ex pleomorphic adenoma 191
 floor of mouth 101
 in situ 141
 larynx, treatment of 147
 tongue 101
Cardiovascular accident 156
Cardiovascular incident 149
Cardiovascular insufficiencies 109
Cardiovascular system 126
Carhart's effect 45
Carhart's notch 45
Carotid artery rupture 204
Carotid bifurcation 12
Carotid canal, identify 144
Cartilage infection 117
Cartilage invasion 136
Cartilaginous, anterior 55
Cartilaginous, junction of 6
Cell, large 16
Cellulitis 5, 6
Central nervous systems disorders 149
Cerebellar dysfunction, tests for 36
Cerebellar function tests 12
Cerebral edema 204
 stage of 32
Cerebrospinal fluid leak 62
Cerebrovascular accidents 127
Cervical
 esophagus 150
 lymph nodes 202
 lymphadenopathy 195
 nodes, treatment of 168
 spine surgery, anterior 118, 126
Chandler's staging 83
Chassaignac's triangle 203
Chemosis 162
Chest, X-ray 76, 88
Choanal atresia 57
Choanal polyps 81
Cholesteatoma 8, 16, 20, 22, 24
Chondroma 67
Chondronecrosis 155
Chondrosarcoma 79
Chordoma 68, 82
Chronic otitis media squamous type, types of 21
Chylous fistula 204
Cochlear fistula 26
Cochlear implants 46
Collagen 128
 vascular disease 127
Colorectal polyposis 69
Commissure, anterior 121
Concha bullosa 65
Concurrent facial palsy, causes of bilateral 29
Conductive hearing loss 9
Congenital nystagmus 39
Congested nasal mucosa 53
Conjunctival edema 162
Constipation 159
Conus elasticus 142
Cord palsies 128
Corners of consternation in neck dissection 203
Cortical mastoidectomy 18
Cottle's test 51
Cough, chronic 117
Cranial nerve function, tests for 36
Craniopharyngioma 82
Cribriform plate 75
Cricoarytenoid joint, arthritis of 116
Cricoid cartilage 143
CSF otorrhea 1
Cushing syndrome 169
Cysts 6, 123
 in tonsil 105

D

da Vinci's surgical robot 147
Dalrymple's sign 162
Deep lamina propria 121
Deformities 5
Dehiscent jugular bulb 8
Dental cysts 183
Dermal collagen 128
Dermatitis 5, 6
Deviated nasal septum 49, 57, 65

Device failure 48
Diabetes 159
mellitus 107, 109
Diabetic neuropathy 4
Direct bony erosion 31
Discovered indirect laryngoscopy 121
Distant metastases 74, 164
Diurnal variation of voice 117
Dix Hallpike maneuver 12, 36
Dizziness 32
Doll's eye manoeuvre 36
Dynamic visual acuity test 36
Dysarthria, causes of 117
Dysphagia 94, 145, 118, 152
Dyspnea 145

E

Ear, examination of 20, 28, 163
Ectopic thyroid 166
Edema 6
Electroglottography 123
Electrogustometry 28
Electromyography 29, 128
Electroneuronography 28
Electronic larynx 144
Electronystagmography 36
Electrophysiological tests 28
Emissary veins 31
Emphysema, surgical 143
Empty nose syndrome 56
Encephalitis signs and symptoms 32
Encephalocele 70
Endoscope 122
Endoscopic dacryocystorhinostomy 63
Endoscopic polypectomy, results of 64
Endotracheal intubation 118
Eosinophilic granuloma 16
Epiglottis 120, 134
Epilepsy 159
Epstein-Barr virus 192
Erythema 5
Esophageal malignancies 125
Esophageal speech 145
Esophagus 118
Ethmoid labyrinth 79
Ethmoid sinus tumors 77
Ethmoids multiple 58
Eustachian tube 26
anatomy of 43
dysfunction 16
functions 42
orifice 8
Exaggerated gag reflex 120
Exophthalmoses 162
Extracapsular dissection of thyroid gland 176
Extracranial meningioma 82
Extradural abscess 31, 32
Eye 30
examination of 72, 81, 162
Eyelid retraction 162

F

Face, examination of 27
Facial nerve 21, 187, 190
branches 204
function, tests for 27
palsy, causes of alternating 29
paralysis 27, 31, 32, 48, 183
causes of recurrent 29
degrees of 29, 30
symptoms of 181
weakness 187
Facial paralysis, causes of 31
Facial recess 24
Failure of cholesteatoma surgery 24
Fallacies in TNM classification in glottic cancer 145
Fallacies of
N staging 201
staging in supraglottic tumors 136
False cords 120, 134, 140
False negative Rinne 9
False positive fistula sign 10
Fatigue 116
Fess, complications of 63
Fever 5
Fibroma 81
Fibro-osseous dysplasia 69
Fibrosarcoma 79
Fibrous dysplasia 67, 69, 82
Fine needle aspiration cytology 109, 167, 173, 185
of neck node 88
Fissures of Santorini 6
Fistula test 8, 10, 21, 28
Flexible endoscope 122
Follicular thyroid cancer 164
Follicular tumors, treatment plan for 168

Foramen lacerum 76
Foramen rotundum 76
Fovea ethmoidalis 75
Fracture and surgical trauma 31
Frey's syndrome 187
Frontal bone, posterior table of 75
Frontal head of occipitofrontalis 27
Frontal process of maxilla 78
Frontal sinus 70, 79
Fukuda stepping test 12
Fundoscopy 12
Fungal sinusitis 62
Furunculosis 4, 6

G

Gardner's syndrome 69
Gastroesophageal reflux disease 118
Gillies fan flap 103
Glasgow hearing aid benefit profile 46
Glomus jugulare 6, 8, 22
Glottal closure 122
Glottic cancer 139, 141, 146
  spread of 142
Glottic incompetence 138
Glottic mass restrict vocal cord mobility 140
Glottis 141
  T staging of 140
Gluck Sorenson's incision 144
Goblet cells 1
Goiter 157, 172
Gorlin's syndrome 70
Grades of pars flaccida retraction 7
Graft necrosis 156
Granular pharyngitis, posterior 53
Granulation tissue 13
Granulomatous lesion 51, 181
  chronic 49, 57
Granulomatous reaction 128
Guillain-Barre's syndrome 29, 127

H

Hair loss 159
Haller cell 65
Hansen's disease 51
Hard of hearing 41
Hard palate, malignancies of 102
Head and neck cancers 131
Head thrust test 11, 36
Headache 50
Hearing loss 4, 41, 159
Heel to toe test 12
Hemangioma 69
Hemangiosarcoma 79
Hemorrhage 156, 157, 204
Hennebert's sign 10, 39
HIV infections 95
Hoarseness of voice 152
Horner's syndrome 85
House Brackman's classification 29
Human papilloma virus 109
Hydroxypatite 128
Hyoepiglottic ligament 135
Hyoid bone 143
Hyperkeratosis 99
Hypertension 50, 107, 109, 159
Hypertrophy 56
  of masseter 182
Hypoanesthesia over face 95
Hypopharyngeal cancer 152, 154
  causes of failure in 156
Hypopharyngeal malignancies 150, 154
Hypopharyngeal tumor
  causes of 153
  symptoms of 152
Hypopharynx, subsites of 151
Hypopharynx, TNM classification for 151
Hypothyroidism 176
  permanent 176
Hypotympanum, parts of 8

I

Iatrogenic cholesteatoma 23
Implants, parts of 46
Inadequate motor function 138
Incisions 78
Incudostapedial joint 8
Indirect laryngoscopy 81, 86, 121, 132, 139, 150, 162, 178
Infected branchial cyst 157
Infection 127
  mononucleosis 29
Inflammation, stage of 32
Inflammatory swelling 181
Influences distant metastasis 145
Infrahyoid epiglottis 121
Infraorbital cell 65
Infraorbital fissure 76
Infratemporal fossa 76

Intermediate lamina propria 121
Internal carotid artery, aberrant 8
Intracranial extension 70, 83
Inverted middle turbinate 65
Inverted papilloma 58, 66-68
Irradiation 114
  blurs margins 92
  complications of 93
Isthmus of thyroid gland 157

J

Juvenile nasopharyngeal angiofibroma 68

K

Kaposi's tumor 95
Keratosis obturans 6
Kero's classification 63
Korner's septum 19

L

Labyrinthitis 10, 31
Lamina propria fatigue 116
Laryngeal cancer 145
  symptoms of 145
Laryngeal nerve
  involvement, causes of superior 127
  paralysis, causes of recurrent 126
Laryngeal stenosis 143
Laryngitis 117
  chronic 146
Laryngocele 157, 178
  external 157
Laryngopharyngeal carcinoma 148
Laryngopharyngeal reflux 118
Laryngopharynx 118
Lateral boundary 135
Left vocal cord paralysis 125
Leukemia 29
Leukoplakia 95, 99
Lid lag 162
Likert scale 53
Lingual thyroid swelling 105
Lip 96
Loop of Galen 176
Loss of sensory innervation 138
Loud sound produces nystagmus 39
Lower limit of supraglottis 134
Lyme's disease 29
Lymph nodes 157, 160, 190
Lymphatic aggregates 105
Lymphatic drainage 75
  of hypopharynx 152
Lymphoepithelioma 110
Lymphoma 110, 192

M

MacEvan's triangle 18
Magnetic resonance imaging 109
Malignant masses 58
Malignant nasal masses 49
Malignant otitis externa 4
Malignant tumors 190
Mandibular tumor 183
Marginal edge edema 124
Marginal mandibular nerve 192
Mastoid infection 16
Mastoid tenderness 9
Mastoidectomy 18, 31
Maxilla, posterior wall of 75
Maxillary malignancies, staging of 73
Maxillary sinus 73
  tumor 76
Maxillary tumors, types of radiotherapy for 77
Maximal forced nasal inspiration 53
Maximal stimulation test 28
Maximum speech reception score 15
Mean pressure 54
Meatoplasty, size of 6
Medial maxillectomy 69
Median labiomandibular glossotomy 155
Medullary carcinoma
  thyroid, types of 168
  treatment plan for 168
Medullary thyroid cancer 165
Melkersson-Rosenthal syndrome 29
Meniere's disease 10, 39
Meningioma 68
Meningitis 5, 31, 32, 48
Menopause 117
Mesotympanum cholesteatoma, posterior 24
Messerklinger and Wigand techniques 62
Metaplasia 22
Microlaryngeal surgery 124
Middle cranial fossa 76
Middle ear
  avascular mass 8
  fluid 8
  protection 43
  tumors 8

Middle latency reflex 44
Midline swellings 157
Migraine 34
Mobility of drum 8
Mobius syndrome 29
Mouth, floor of 96, 101
Mucocele 70
Mucoepidermoid carcinoma 191
Mucoid nasal discharge 66
Mucosa over promontory 8
Mucosal chronic otitis media, types of 13
Multicellular theory 188
Multiple cranial nerve palsies 4
Multiple sclerosis 127
Muscle fatigue 116
  abdominal 116
Muscle tension dysphonia 129
Myasthenia gravis 116, 127
Myocardial infarction 156
Myoepithelioma 183, 186
Myringoplasty 17
  complications of 17

N

Nasal allergy, tests for 53
Nasal block 49, 50, 66
Nasal bone 78
Nasal cavity
  and ethmoid sinus, T staging of 73
  subsites of 74
Nasal cycle 55
Nasal diptheria 49
Nasal discharge 49
Nasal endoscopy 75
Nasal obstruction visual analog scale 53
Nasal septum 79
Nasal surgery 51
Nasal valve 51, 56
Nasopharyngeal angiofibroma 50, 80, 82, 84
  origin of 82
Nasopharyngeal carcinoma 85, 87, 88, 90
Nasopharyngeal mass 57
Nasopharynx 76, 83
  biopsy, examination of 88
  malignancies of 50
Neck dissection 98, 203
  classify 115
  complications of 204
  comprehensive 203
Neck muscle fatigue 116
Neck nodes 136, 152
Neck swellings in 106, 145, 189
Neck, examination of 86, 96, 108, 121, 132, 150, 160
Neck, ultrasound of 166
Neoplasia of temporal bone 26
Neoplasm 5
Nerve
  excitability test 28
  injury 204
  paralysis, classify 127
Neural involvement, symptoms of 181
Neuroma 68
  of facial nerve 183
Neuropraxia 127
Nodal metastasis 201
Non-iatrogenic trauma 127
Noninfected branchial cyst 157
Non-recurrent laryngeal nerve 128
Non-steroidal anti-inflammatory drug 59
Non-surgical methods of relieving deafness 46
Nose
  and paranasal sinuses, malignancies of 49
  and peripheral nervous system, CT scan of 64
  and PNS, examination of 12, 96
  examination of 182
  external 58, 66, 81

O

Obstructs frontal sinus 65
Odisoft rhino 54
Odontogenic ameloblastoma 68
Odontogenic keratocyst 70
Odontogenic cysts 69
Odynophagia 94, 118
Ohngren's line 76
Olfactory fossa 63
Oncocytoma 183, 186
Onodi cells 65
Opacification, complete 62
Ophthalmoplegia 162
Optokinetic nystagmus 35, 36
Oral cancer 96
Oral cavity 81, 94, 190
  carcinoma 99

examination of 72, 86, 95, 162
malignancies 98
Oral leukoplakia 95
Oral tongue 96
Orbicularis oculi 27
Orbicularis oris 27
Orbital apex 76
Orbital complications 63
Orbital erosion 70
Oropharyngeal malignancies 109, 112
Oropharyngeal mass 105
Oropharynx 72, 86, 111
examination of 96, 162
Orthopantogram 98
Ossicular chain, parts of 13
Ossiculoplasty 25
Oscillopsia 39, 40
Osteogenic sarcoma 79
Osteoma 67, 69, 82
Otalgia 1, 145, 152
Otitis media 4
acute 4, 16
chronic 1, 20, 21, 23
Otomycosis 4
Overhanging epiglottis 120

P

Pain 1, 183
absence of 133
Painful swellings 157
Painless otorrhea 32
Palatal mass 102
Palatal tumors 69
Palate 96
Pale middle ear mucosa 32
Papillary carcinoma, treatment plan for 167
Papilloma 81, 146
Paraglottic space 135
Parakeratosis 99
Paralysis of
recurrent nerve, permanent 176
superior laryngeal nerves, permanent 176
Parapharyngeal tumors 157
Parathyroid neoplastic syndromes 169
Parkinson's disease 127
Parotid gland 186
inflammatory lesions of 186
Parotid malignancy, signs of 183
Parotid swelling 180
Parotidectomy
complications of 187
types of 188
Partial pharyngectomy 155
Peak nasal inspiration flow 53
Perichondritis of thyroid cartilage 157
Perilabyrinthine osteitis, chronic 26
Perilymph fistula 10
Petrositis 31
Petrous apex cholesteatoma 26
Pharyngeal pouch 118, 157
Pharyngeal wall, posterior 150
Pharyngectomy 156
Pharyngotomy, lateral 112, 155
Photoglottography 123
Phrenic nerve 204
Plasmacytoma 79
Pleomorphic adenoma 183, 186
Plummer-Vinson's syndrome 95
Pneumatic otoscopy, uses of 8
Pneumothorax 204
Polymorphic low grade carcinoma 191
Polyostotic fibrous dysplasia 70
Polypoidal mucosal thickening 62
Polyposis 62
Polyps 13, 59
Polytetrafluoroethylene 128
Positive fistula test 10
Postaural abscess 31
Postcricoid irradiation 155
Postcricoid region 150
Posterior margin 7
Postnasal drip 53
Post-stapedectomy 10
Postural balance, examination of 38
Posturography 36
Preauricular lymphadenitis 183
Preauricular region 5
Pre-epiglottic space 135
Pressure equalization 43
Primary tumor 164
Profuse pale granulation 32
Proteus mirabalis 13
Pseudostratified ciliated columnar epithelium 1
Pterygoid canal 76
Pterygomaxillary fissure 76, 78
Pterygopalatine fossa 75
Pulmonary diseases tuberculosis 109
Pulmonary metastasis 109
Pulsatile swelling 196

Pure tone audiometry 14, 41
Pyriform fossa 120, 140, 150
  apex of 121
  mass 153
  tumors 152

Q

Quadrangular membrane 135

R

Rabies 29
Radiation induced laryngeal edema 155
Radical mastoidectomy 26
Radical neck dissection 203
  extended 203
Radicular cyst 69
Radioiodine therapy 171
  contraindications for 171
Radiotherapy 100, 101
  complications of 154
Radkowski's classification 83
Recurrent cholesteatoma 6
Recurrent laryngeal nerve
  neuropathy in diabetes 127
  paralysis 129
Recurrent pleomorphic adenoma 193
Referred otalgia 94, 149
Referred pain 1
Regional lymph node 74,, 164, 183
Regurgitation of food 118
Reinke's edema 124
Reinke's space 124, 142
Relative loudness test 9
Remove inferior turbinate 55
Renal system 4
Repeat radiotherapy 92
Respiratory
  failure 156
  system 126
Retraction pockets 8
Retraction, signs of 7
Retromolar trigone 96, 108
Rhinomanometry 53
Rhinoscopy
  anterior 51, 72
  posterior 52, 72
Rhinosinusitis 57
Rhinosporidiosis 50
Right nasal cavity 72
Right recurrent laryngeal nerve 176
Rinne's test 10
Robotic thyroidectomy 177
Role of HRCT 29
Romberg's
  sign 21
  test 12, 36
Rosenmüller, fossa of 90
Rotation test 37, 36, 38

S

Saccades 35
Saccular functions 39
Salivary flow test 28
Salivary gland 180, 186
  neoplasia, theories of 188
  scintigraphy 185
  tumor 79, 82, 110
    TNM classification for 193
Salivary tumors, common 186
Salvage surgery 92
Sarcoidosis 29
Schirmer's test 28
Schwartz's mastoidectomy 18
Scintigraphy 166
Sebaceous cyst 182
Secondary neck nodes 157
Semicircular canal fistula, lateral 10
Sensitive test 10
Sensorineural loss 9
  after mastoidectomy, causes of 26
Septal deviation, types of 55
Septoplasty 54
Sessile swelling 124
Session's classification 83
Sialography 185
Simple mastoidectomy 18
Sinonasal
  malignancy 71, 73
  mass 87
  polyps 57
Sinus disease, role of MRI in 62
Sinus thrombophlebitis, lateral 31
Sinus thrombosis, lateral 5, 32
Sinus tympanic 24
Sinusitis, acute 62
Sinusoidal test 38
Sistrunk's operation 179
Sjogren's syndrome 192
Skull base erosion 70
Skull base osteomyelitis 6

Skull based osteomylitis 22
Smaller supraglottic tumors 137
Smooth pursuit 35
Soft tissue 56
Sore throat 152
Speech audiometry 15
Sphenoid sinus 75, 83
Sphenopalatine foramen 76
Spiral cord 115
Spontaneous nystagmus 37
Spread of infection, routes of 31
Squamous cell carcinoma 79, 95, 110, 146, 192
  of vocal cord 146
Squamous epithelium 121
Squamous otitis media, active 22
Stage angiofibroma 83
Stage oral cavity malignancies 97
Stage supraglottic tumors 134
Stapedectomy, contraindications for 46
Stapedial reflex 28
Staphylococcus aureus 13
Stellwag's sign 162
Stenosis 6
Stereotaxic radiotherapy 92
Sternomastoid muscle, identify medial border of 144
Stimulation of facial nerve 48
Stridor 118, 145
Stroboscopic light source 122
Stylomastoid foramen 28
Subacute thyroiditis 157
Subdural abscess 31, 32
Subglottic region 121
Subglottic tumors, behavior of 146
Subhyoid bursitis 157
Subluxation of incus 19
Submandibular gland
  benign swelling of 190
  resection 192
  swelling 189
Superficial lamina propria 121
Superficial parotidectomy 187, 188
Superior laryngeal nerve paralysis
  signs of 127
  symptoms of 127
Superior semicircular canal dehiscence 5
Supernumerary teeth 69
Suppurative lymph nodes 157
Supraclavicular region 91
Supracricoid larygectomy 143
Supraglottic carcinoma 130
Supraglottic laryngectomy 138
  contraindications for 137
Supraglottic tumors 133
  spread 134
  symptoms of 133
Suprahyoid pharyngotomy 112
Surgical excision of mass, contraindications for 78
Swallowing liquids 149
Swelling exactly 106
Swelling, relation of 196
Swellings, lateral 157
Syphilis 10, 107

T

Temporomandibular joint disease 1
Temporal bone 115
Temporalis fascia 16
Thermal injury 126
Thoracic surgery 118, 126
Thornwaldt's and mucosal cysts 81
Threshold comparison test 9
Thyroglossal cyst 157, 178, 179
Thyroglottic ligament 142
Thyrohyoid membrane 135
Thyroid
  cancer
    prognosis of 171
    TNM staging for 164
  gland invasion 136
  lateral lobe of 157
  neoplasm 157
  nodule 157
  scan 166
  surgery 118, 126, 177
Thyroidectomy 170
Thyroiditis, acute 157
Thyrotoxicosis 162
TNM staging 97
Tongue 113
  movement, abnormality of 189
  posterior third of 120
Tonsil and pharyngeal wall 113
Total conservative 188
Total laryngectomy 77, 144, 156
Total maxillectomy 77
Total pharyngectomy 155
Tracheal necrosis 156

Tracheoesophageal shunt 145
Transglottic tumor 133
Transhyoid pharyngotomy
  anterior 155
  lateral 155
Transitional cell carcinoma 79
Traumatic facial nerve palsy 30
Treat empty nose syndrome 56
Treat lip cancer 103
True cords 120, 140
Tuberculosis 4, 16, 107, 133, 146, 160, 186
  otitis media 32
Tuberculous lymph nodes 157
Tuberculous otitis media 22
Tullio phenomenon 39
Tumor 16, 70
  histopathology of 146
  necrosis factor 59
  of oral cavity, common 100
  of parotid gland, common malignant 190
  of submandibular salivary gland, common malignant 190
  volume 136
Tuning fork test 28
Turbinate hypertrophy 57
Tympanic membrane 8, 21, 28
Tympanometry 41
Tympanosclerosis 8
Tympanostomy tubes 16

U

Ultrasound glottography 123
Unilateral choanal atresia 49
Unterberger's test 12, 36
Upper lip defects 103
Upper respiratory tract infection 117

V

Vagus nerve 152
Vallate papillae 105
Vallecula 120
Velocity step test 38
Ventricle 121, 134
Ventricular band 134
Verrucous carcinoma 146
Vertical partial laryngectomy 143
Vertigo 34
  peripheral and central 39
Vestibular evoke myogenic potential test 36
Vestibular function, tests for 10
Vestibulo-ocular reflex 35, 36
Vestibulo-oculomotor reflex 35
Vibratory margin of cord, scarring of 116
Vocal cord
  pace maker 129
  palsy 152
Vocal fatigue 116
Vocal fold paralysis 116
Vocal ligament 142
Vocal nodules 116
Vocal sulcus 123
Voice alteration, causes of 129
Vomiting 159
von Graefe's sign 162

W

Walled abscess, stage of 32
Wallerian degeneration 28, 29, 127
Warthin's tumor 183, 186
Wegener's granuloma 22
Whitish debris 6
Whitish flakes 21
Wound infection 204